In Good Company

In Good Company

An Escort's Guide

Kay Good

First published in 2005 by Fusion Press,
a division of Satin Publications Ltd.
101 Southwark Street
London SE1 0JF
UK
info@visionpaperbacks.co.uk
www.visionpaperbacks.co.uk
Publisher: Sheena Dewan

A catalogue record for this book is available from the British Library.

ISBN: 1-904132-71-5

2 4 6 8 10 9 7 5 3 1

Cover and text design by ok?design
Printed and bound in the UK by Mackays of Chatham Ltd,
Chatham, Kent

Contents

Acknowledgements   ix

Legal Disclaimer   x

Introduction   1

Chapter One: Getting Started   22

Chapter Two: Clients   38

Chapter Three: The Reality of Escorting   63

Chapter Four: A Day in the Life of . . .   96

Chapter Five: Other Forms of Sex Work   116

Chapter Six: The Media and the Law   157

Chapter Seven: A Guide for Clients   187

Chapter Eight: Making the Most of Being an Escort   205

The Checklist   215

Resources   219

References   240

About the Author   245

This book is for Ella,
whose love and inspiration
enabled this book to be written.

And for all GRRLS everywhere.

Acknowledgements

I would like to thank all the people, sex workers and people outside the industry, who contributed to putting this book together. You know who you are. For their support and advice I would particularly like to thank Ella, Delaney Martin, Katy, Natalie, Kim in Australia, Kim in London, Kye Lockwood, Zak Jane Keir, Gemma, Shirley, Kat, Nicki, Robin, Sharon, Zoe, Mistress Anna, Britta, Katya, Marit and Kiwi Alan.

For their advice and their tireless campaigning for all women I would like to thank the ECP, the effervescent Dr Tuppy Owens and The Outsiders Group.

For starting all this off I have to thank Emily Dubberley and Sheena Dewan.

For her friendship, research, baths and dinners too numerous to count, I want to thank Fiona Daly.

Last but not least thank you to Chris Watts for the support, criticism, love and tolerance that enabled this book to happen.

Legal Disclaimer

The author and the publishers in no way wish to encourage anyone to enter the sex industry.

This book has been written solely as a guide and advice for anyone thinking of entering the industry. It is also written as a guide and advice for anyone already in the industry who may be unaware of their legal and social position within the industry and the state.

The legal status of sex workers varies from country to country so it is up to the reader to establish the legal boundaries that exist in his or her own state and act accordingly.

Neither the author nor the publisher condones illegal activities of any kind.

This book has been written solely to impart information. In no way is its intent to lure people into, or glamorise, the sex industry.

The author and publisher are providing readers with this information so that they may have the opportunity to make informed choices on a subject that is surrounded by misinformation and myth.

The author and the publishers do not condone drug use of any kind and any references to drug use and abuse only reflect an honest account of everyday society, particularly within the sex industry.

Introduction

In Good Company is primarily a guide to escorting. It is designed to answer every question that might occur to anyone thinking of escorting, anyone currently struggling with more 'difficult' forms of prostitution and even just the curious. It covers everything from getting started, finding the right agency, clients, money, relationships, current social attitudes, the practical day-to-day realities, the law, media, other forms of sex work and working as an independent.

Second, self-respect is a theme that comes up many times in this book because it is so important to have it, whatever you do in your life. Without self-respect the world will exploit and use you. With it you can do almost anything. *In Good Company* is an affirmation to all women that we have the right to do what we want with our bodies and our lives.

Third, it contains a section that should be read by all men wishing to use the services of an escort which sets out in very plain language how one goes about finding, hiring and treating escorts.

Finally, there is a comprehensive resources section at the end listing help and support services in most of the cities mentioned in this book.

Many people, a lot of them women, have written about sex, sexuality and the sex industry. From pornography to feminism, from the internet to women's magazines, we have been bombarded with what we should think, feel and be. Make up your own mind. The contributions and case studies in this book are all true. Some are humorous. Some are horrific. They were all written by real women, and one or two men, from their own real life experiences – all I have done is correct the grammar (where it was appropriate), clean up the spelling and change the identities. Because these contributions are real they are worth taking seriously. The advice that they and I give comes from cumulative years of experience.

I have dipped in and out of the adult industries most of my working life, in one form or another. As an 18-year-old new arrival in London with no money, after being contacted by an acquaintance in the Australian television industry who pointed out that I could solve a few of my current problems in this way, I 'worked' the hotel bars. I didn't do it for long – for about three to five months – as I was in love, but it did sort out some of the tight economic scrapes I found myself in. Throughout my twenties I was a glamour model. When I was in my twenties and early thirties I did

Introduction

text and phone sex to supplement my income. In my late thirties I went to work in a dungeon, ran someone else's escort agency and met lots and lots of sex workers. I became appalled by the stories of women who had suffered corruption, exploitation and abuse. I realised the way to promote change was to create a different working example. With the backing of other sex workers GoodGrrls came into being. It is an escort agency designed, cultivated and promoted on the basis of intelligent women making intelligent choices and interacting on a business level with intelligent men without violence or coercion.

GoodGrrls became a success because, firstly, the clients who use the agency know that they will get exactly what they want, and that what they see is what they get. And, secondly, because the women who approach me, many having heard of me through word of mouth, know that they are safe and have somewhere they can get advice and support should they need it.

With the right agency, escorting can be a legitimate and safe form of sex work – the parameters are stated before meeting, the client is checked for authenticity and the agent is, ideally, although not always, watching your back from a distance should anything go wrong. But there are many different forms of sex work and I intend to address them all – street prostitution, domination, text and phone sex, stripping and lap dancing, porn and glamour modelling. How you treat yourself and others, and what your own personal parameters are, is up to you. But know that the choice should always be yours. If you make the decision to work within the sex industry do so from an informed point of view. You can be what the law defines as a 'common prostitute' and work the streets coked off your face giving the bulk of your money to a man. Or you can have a little dignity, become an escort and, with good sense and hard work, make a decent living for yourself.

Escorting can mean many things but the essence of what you are selling is time for money – and for 99 per cent of that time that means sex for money. For many people hiring escorts it is also about participating in someone else's youth and beauty – for an aging man to spend time in the company of a beautiful young woman can be the physical and psychological tonic that gives him a renewed lease of life. A few people hire escorts literally just for company – to be a friend, to listen without judgement and to empathise with that person's needs, whether they are emotional, psychological or sexual.

Escorting is in fact quite an honest way to earn money when one looks at how we as women get through life. Any adult woman who intelligently assesses the sexual interaction she has had with men throughout her life will discover that on at least one occasion she will have 'bartered' her sexual favours or used her sexuality to some extent for personal gain – whether that be from simply getting a man to carry your suitcase, buy you a drink or get you off a parking ticket, to getting promotion, dinner and a cab home, a piece of jewellery, a new bathroom or a holiday (most of which I myself have done). Or, at a more basic level, for the money to put food in her fridge or to feed her child. We make these transactions as wives, lovers and employees. So what is the difference between that and escorting? Although many people will not perceive a wife denying her husband sex till he gets the new bathroom sorted or the single mother who has sex with a 'friend' so he can pay this month's electricity bill for her as being sex work, it is still a form of prostitution and it is still using our bodies to get what we want from someone else. At least with escorting we are being honest about what we are trading our bodies and time for – money. As the English Collective of Prostitutes (ECP) has said:

> Money comes into everything – it shouldn't but it does, because that's the kind of society we live in. Money determines how you are treated, it determines where you live, it determines what kind of police protection you get, it determines what school, what education – everything is determined by what your income is. Money determines all our relationships. But relationships in general are not seen like that. They are seen as psychological, nothing to do with economics. But when it comes to prostitution nobody can avoid the fact that there is an economic transaction going on and that the woman is definitely doing it for the money – that's what she gets for it. It's the same all over. It's just that when it comes to prostitution it's clear, the cards are on the table. And that's why many men like going to prostitutes, because there's no involvement, you know exactly what the

transaction is, you don't have to pretend to be in love, you don't have to pretend to be interested, you don't have to pretend all these things. It is in that sense a cleaner relationship.[1]

We live in a society that disables us from having the things we need and want while dangling the advertising carrot over us at every opportunity. A society that pushes debt and credit at us from such an early age that many graduates never recover from the financial mess they get into by achieving their degrees, and many young mothers and their children never rise above the poverty line. On the 1 December 2004 The Joseph Rowntree Foundation and the National Policy Institute reported that there were '3.6 million children and 3.9 million working-aged adults without children living below the British government's "poverty line" in 2002/2003.'[2] According to the US Census, there were 35.9 million people in America living in poverty in 2003, up 1.3 million from 2002.[3] And in Australia unemployment in April 2005 increased to 540,900.[4]

Escorting gives women the chance to rise above mundane, soul-destroying, badly paid existences and gain a lot of the things society tells us we should aspire to – the mortgaged 'nice' roof over our heads, the clothing that labels us as a success, the wherewithal to get a cab home and, more importantly, it gives us the ability to be able to pay for it ourselves.

Ideally, if nothing else, on having read this book you will be able to decide whether escorting, or indeed any form of sex work, is right for you. Don't believe everything you hear – investigate for yourself, do your research and don't make yourself a victim. All forms of work have their up sides and their down – make sure that whatever you do is right for you. Don't do anything just because someone tells you to. If you can avoid it, don't do anything that makes you unhappy, whether the field is the sex industry or working in McDonald's.

Reasons to escort and reasons not to escort

I sometimes advertise for escorts in women's magazines. Many of the women who phone me for an interview have hung on to that magazine for months on the basis of 'Maybe I will, maybe I won't. Let's see how bad things can really get before I phone that number.' More often than not for most women it is a case of drastic solutions to drastic situations.

At some time in our lives many of us find that we simply do not have enough money to survive. This is the primary reason that most people go into sex work. There are other reasons – sexual stimulation, a financial goal, to escape a violent parent or partner, or a psychological kick – but the truth is most people do it because they need the money. The psychological implications of all sex work are vast. If you are not a stable person in good mental health – and be honest with yourself about this – I suggest you try every other option open to you before embarking on a life in the sex industry. Thinking that because you are a natural submissive the next logical step is to become a whore is patently not healthy. While it can be a stimulating and invigorating way to earn a living it can also make you very tired, expose you to sides of life you may not be familiar with and, for many people, it goes hand in hand with some major and possibly painful life changes as many of the case studies in this book show.

Reasons to escort

Your sexuality

Many women, as we can see on the internet in particular, have come out radically in declaring their sexuality with pride. They are sexy and sexual. They want to pick their men, dictate how they express their sexuality and predominantly don't wish to be burdened with a relationship afterwards. For these women escorting is the perfect career. If you love sex – I mean genuinely love sex – then doing the thing you love most in the world and getting paid for it is a unique buzz. Take the example of Minnie, who made her own choices sensibly:

> I worked in restaurants for most of the time until I was 26. I knew from this work that I had the ability to make men buy me things. If I wanted a new dress or a piece of jewellery I had only to mention it and, hey, my charm and their gullibility ensured I would get it. I decided to take the next step and start charging for my time. I began by joining an agency where I learnt the ropes of the business,

Introduction

and when I felt confident enough I became an independent. I can earn up to £1,000 a day – I own my own home and rent another, I'm saving for my retirement in the not too distant future and I have several lovers. More to the point, I'm a sex addict. From the time I started having sex I knew I was, well, insatiable. My boyfriends couldn't keep up with me and I was always playing away just to get the amount of sexual attention I needed. This way I get the best of it all. I have travelled extensively, met some amazing and wonderful people and I am totally financially independent.

Minnie's case is not unique. Sam was a married university graduate working for the government:

I got into escorting through experimenting with my sexuality with my husband. We both loved sex and had decided to further our experimentation by going to swingers parties. I loved it so much that soon after I talked to my husband and we agreed I would set up an apartment in the city and work five days a week as an escort. As long as weekends were my husband's we would be fine. I found myself a luxury apartment and went into business. I hated my previous job, it was boring and futile. I love sex, plus I earn up to $1,800 per day. This life has its drawbacks but it also has its advantages!

In Good Company

Safe sex should always be practised at swingers parties.

Your financial situation

Getting into financial difficulty is nothing new. In the UK, at the time of writing, the average household debt is approximately £7,664 excluding mortgages and £44,818 including mortgages.[5] In Australia, 5.1 per cent of the population in April 2005 was registered unemployed.[6] And women earn, on average, about 10 per cent less than men.'[7]

I don't know about you but I find these figures very scary – with so many people living that close to the edge financially, it amazes me that there are not more people working in industries such as ours. It is no wonder that most of the women who approach my agency do so because they are in a financial bind. They are either in debt, have something they really want the money for – like a car, travel or a breast job – or they are students or single mums (more on them later).

Escorting can be a good solution. But make sure it is the right choice of solution for you. Can you be an escort and not have it interfere with your day-to-day existence? Lovers and 'day job' employers are unlikely to understand why you need to escort, no matter what your situation. They just won't. Being an escort is a double life, and being single-minded and a good actress like Annie can help:

> I am a make-up artist, have a boyfriend, and I escorted for three months. I managed it by breaking my life up into mutually exclusive boxes. I worked in a department store during the day,

escorted Monday, Wednesday and Thursday nights – my boyfriend thought I was doing a course – and the rest of the evenings I spent with him. When he played football on Sundays I sometimes escorted as well. I did this from September through to December and then gave my family the best Christmas ever – I took them all to the Caribbean! I don't think I'll do it again, but it was something I had been curious about doing for a long time. Once I did it though the 'mystique' definitely disappeared.

Students

Over the years I have worked with many student escorts. It can be an ideal way to get through a university degree, although I recommend stopping escorting during exam time – the stress factor is too high! Many students leave university with a colossal debt, owing money to banks, parents and friends. British graduates owed an average of £12,180 in 2004, according to a study by NatWest bank. The study also found that 2005's new students 'expect they will need £26,000 to pay for their time at college'[8]. In America 25.9 per cent of all white bachelor's degree recipients in 2000 graduated with over $25,000 debt and 29.5 per cent of all black bachelor's degree recipients graduated with over $25,000 debt.[9] In Australia it is estimated that the cost of undertaking the necessary degree to become a registered dental practitioner will be in the vicinity of $130,000 to $150,000 for full fee-paying students.[10]

In Good Company

Many students, being away from home for the first time, find the conditions of renting and social freedom too much of a whirl to realise just how much debt they are getting themselves into, and banks and governments encourage this state of financial fantasy. Escorting is a way to not become a victim of your own education, as Hannah found:

> I was halfway through my medical degree when I realised that my debts were making me more and more depressed. I tried Prozac, but I was still in debt. I tried counselling, but that meant I was even more in debt. Then I tried escorting. Within a year I had reduced my bank loans from £13,000 to £1,500. I continued escorting until I got my degree and I am now a practicing doctor in a large teaching hospital. When I began my internship I had no debt, the money to pay my rent for a year and the ability to buy lots of nice new clothes. I was determined not to become one of the graduate debt statistics, but it was the hardest thing I ever had to do. I live in terminal fear that I will come across an ex-client on the wards!

Single mothers

If you are desperate to keep your kids fed and clothed and give them all the other things they need and want, then escorting can be a good way to achieve this. You can work when you and your children's schedules permit. You can dictate your own hours. If you have a good babysitting network no one need ever know what you are doing. In Britain an unemployed lone mother with one child receives £81.23 a week as an asylum seeker and £113.87 as a UK resident after rent and council benefits. (That's less than half an hour's time with a client for a £250-per-hour escort.) In Australia a single woman with child receives $426.90 per fortnight. In America the basic SSI (Social Security Income) payment, as of January 2005, is $579 per month for an eligible individual (half a day's work for a successful New York escort).[11]

Reasons not to escort

Coercion

Some parts of the world however have it worse off than those living at the lowest levels in the UK, USA and Australia, and it seems that it is generally women who are the first victims of economic or social tragedy. Economic hardship has forced many Eastern European women to London and Paris particularly to work in the sex industry, where one night's work can be the equivalent of a month's pay back home. In Russia:

> Often women with families are forced to work because of insufficient state child allowances and unemployment benefits. Economic hardship has driven some women into prostitution. In the Soviet period, prostitution was viewed officially as a form of social deviancy that was dying out as the Soviet

Union advanced toward communism. In the 1990s, organised crime has become heavily involved in prostitution, both in Russia and in the cities of Central and Western Europe, to which Russian women are often lured by bogus advertisements for match-making services or modelling agencies. According to one estimate, 10,000 women from Central Europe, including a high proportion of Russians, have been lured or forced into prostitution in Germany alone.[12]

Many people end up in the sex industry not by their own choosing. This is, of course, completely wrong. No human being in the world has the right to tell you what to do with your own body. No one has the right to own you or dictate what you do with your time or your money. If you find yourself in this situation, get out immediately! Call the police and/or tell someone who is not involved (see the resources section at the end of this book for useful contacts for support groups and agencies).

There are very few accurate statistics that can be relied upon regarding the international trading of people for sex work. Undoubtedly it does go on.

However you don't have to be trafficked across international borders to end up in sex work for reasons not of your own choosing. Being emotionally, mentally or physically pushed towards any form of sex work by another person is the best reason *not* to do it. If your partner suggests it and says it would turn him or her on, then you should seriously think

Introduction

about replacing them. If you feel you want to play the submissive whore, then role play it with your partner. Do not take the actual step of entering the sex industry to further the game – more often than not it will ruin your relationship and cause you mental pain. If you or your partner need the money for drug addiction problems, yours or theirs, seek qualified professional help (see resources).

Going escorting for someone else's dependencies is a waste of time, energy and love. Going escorting to feed your own drug addiction is self-destroying and self-defeating. There is no point escorting if you are not 100 per cent confident about who you are and what you want. It should be a choice and not an emotional gun to the head. Melissa's story shows why:

> I met Judith when I was 14, she was the most amazing thing and I would have done anything for her. I ran away from home so we could live together. By the time I was 16 and she was 18 she had a full-on drug habit. She would take anything anyone gave her and the more she took the more she wanted. She sent me out to escort to pay for it all. We both knew it was illegal because I was 16 but she didn't care and I was frightened of losing her so I did it. Eventually she had me hooked on crack and I didn't care how many guys I had sex with. It took me three years to get away from her and off the drugs.

Melissa was underage. It is illegal to escort in the UK until you are 18 years old. Judith was effectively pimping, or profiting from the earnings of Melissa, which is illegal, as well as patently wrong. Both were drug users, which is a dangerous and stupid way of existing within the sex industry.

Revenge

They say revenge is sweet. In my experience this is rarely the case. Going into prostitution to 'pay someone back' for mistreatment of you is short-sighted to say the least.

Becoming an escort will not make the boyfriend/husband who dumped you come back or make him feel bad about what he has done, as Rachel's story shows:

> I was in love with this guy called Ken but he was married. We had known each other intimately at school but drifted apart. I met up with him again several years later and the spark, the chemistry, was still very much there. We made love on that first meeting. Then he told me he was married. I was completely gutted till he told me that he didn't really love his wife and had been forced into the marriage by their parents. He told me he would leave her. He kept telling me for four years that he loved only me and that he would leave her. Towards the end I started to go crazy, we fought all the time about when and if he was going to leave her. I threatened to go out escorting to prove I didn't need him or his financial support. He laughed in

> my face. So I did it. I wish I hadn't. I haven't seen
> Ken since the day he found out about me seeing
> clients, he just upped and left.

Similarly, becoming an escort will not make the family who abused you recognise that abuse and make amends for it. In fact either of these scenarios is likely to send you to a place that is even worse for your total well-being, as later case studies will show.

Escape

I have met many women over the years who fell into escorting and prostitution as a means of getting away from violent husbands, partners or fathers. Many women find themselves trapped with violent men because they do not have an independent income and are reliant on those men to feed and clothe their children. In 2002, the Women's Aid Federation of England found that '1 in 4 women experience domestic violence over their lifetimes and between 6–10 per cent of women suffer domestic violence in a given year.'[13] The 2001–02 British Crime Survey found that 'there were an estimated 635,000 incidents of domestic violence in England and Wales. Repeat victimisation is common . . . more than half (57 per cent) of victims of domestic violence are involved in more than one incident. No other type of crime has a rate of repeat victimisation as high.'[14]

Every minute in the UK, the police receive a call from the public for assistance in a case of domestic violence.

In Good Company

They receive an estimated 1,300 calls each day and over 570,000 each year.[15] For further information on the British Crime Surveys, a separate briefing is available from Women's Aid.[16]

According to the American Institute on Domestic Violence, 'every 9 seconds a woman is beaten in the United States. Between 3 and 4 million women are battered each year. 85–95 per cent of all domestic violence victims are female.'[17] And in New Zealand domestic violence is a major social problem, estimated to cost the nation between 1.187 billion and 5.302 billion dollars per year.[18]

I do not recommend escorting or prostitution as a way out of a domestically violent environment, but it has helped some women escape the trap of having to go back to violent partners once they have escaped, as Lucy explains:

> I was living with a man and my son by a previous partner. It started out fine but after a year he started bullying both my son Matthew and me. By the end of the second year he had broken four of my ribs, given me a permanent scar above my left eye and totally broken my confidence. The worst of it all was that Matthew saw almost everything. I left this man three times but I couldn't cope without the financial support. I have no family who would help me. Eventually, I ran into an old acquaintance in a supermarket and she told me about a place she was working at and said that Matthew and I could stay with her till we got ourselves sorted out. I

worked for six months in that brothel, saved enough money for the deposit on a flat on the other side of London, joined a reputable escort agency and I have not looked back. I am now happily married to a wonderful man with two more gorgeous kids. My time in the brothel was hard but not as bad as living with my ex.

If you are suffering from domestic violence of any kind get help immediately. No one has the right to hurt or intimidate another individual. Go to the police or a refuge, of which there are over 250 in England, Scotland, Wales and Northern Ireland[19] or use any of the resources listed at the back of this book. Jennifer's story is tragic but relevant:

> I was sexually and physically assaulted by my father from the time I was seven. My mother ignored it and eventually left me with him. I ran away at the age of 13. I lived on the streets for a few years and then I got involved in prostitution. I figured if it was all right for my father to have me it was all right for me to sell the same on. After all, I'm damaged goods – who gives a damn?

Don't fall into this trap. Whatever damage occurs to you at the hands of someone else is no reason to enter the sex industry. The best-case result of doing so is that you will survive, block out the memories and never heal the damage.

The worst case is that you will become more screwed up and mentally unstable than you were at the hands of your domestic tormentor.

The Cash Reality

Escorting can make you great money but you have to work at it. Be under no illusions. It rarely happens that a woman just lands onto the sex industry scene in any country and creates such a furore that she becomes instantly rich over night.

There are an estimated 80,000 working prostitutes in the UK.[20] In Holland there are 25,000.[21] In America the National Task Force on Prostitution suggests that over 1 million people in the US have worked as prostitutes – or about 1 per cent of American women.[22] In New Zealand the majority of the 6,000–8,000 prostituted women are Asians. In Auckland, of 4,000 prostituted 800 are Thai, and 400 other Asian women.[23]

Japan has the largest sex industry market for Asian women. There are 'over 150,000 non-Japanese women involved in prostitution, mostly Thai and Filipino women . . . The sex industry accounts for 1 per cent of GNP and equals the country's defence budget.'[24]

The economic collapse of countries like Albania means that 100,000 young women from that country have been trafficked to brothels abroad. Other countries rely on sex tourism. In Thailand, estimates of women in prostitution range from 300,000 to 2.8 million, of which a third are minors and children.[25] All these figures could possibly be a very conservative estimate, no one knows for sure, but that is a hell of a lot of competition.

You can work yourself out of debt and acquire the extra things in life you think you need or want by joining a reputable agency or – when you are experienced enough – by becoming an independent, but to achieve this requires hard work and discipline. The sad truth is that most women do not make lots of money primarily because they spend it as fast as they earn it.

The next chapter describes how to get started. Always remember, if any of this makes you think, 'Oh, no, this is not for me!' then stick with that. Your own instinct is what keeps you alive, listen to it always.

Chapter One

Getting Started

So either your back is against some metaphoric financial wall or you just fancy getting into the industry for a kick – how do you get started?

Undoubtedly the best way to start escorting is with a personal introduction. If you happen to know someone already involved in the industry and can talk to him or her, do so. And if you don't feel comfortable about how your friend is describing the work, or if you feel they're pushing you into it, steer clear. However, by the very nature of the work we do, it is unlikely you will know if you have a friend in the industry. Most escorts keep their working and personal lives totally separate.

You do not have to be a 'classic' kind of gorgeous. People like different things. Men are not just attracted to glamour model lookalikes, just as women are not only attracted to big, hunky Latino types. You do not have to be the world's greatest lover but you can learn from your experience all the time (as Mya's story at the end of this chapter shows).

Getting Started

Thousands of men every day all over the world pay for sex. Their tastes and desires are as varied as your own.

As far as escorting goes (I will deal with other forms of sex work in Chapter Five) the next best place to start is the internet. Go to www.google.com, type in 'escort agency' and your city or area and see what comes up. Look at as many as you can. Closely. Look at the way the women are represented. Look at the rates being charged. Look at the services being offered. Compare all these things with your own image of yourself – do you feel that you can compete with what is already out there? What do you want to earn? Are the rates being charged similar to that figure? And what are you prepared to do for it? Be honest with yourself.

Make a list of all the agencies you like the look of, if any, along with their phone numbers and a contact name if there is one. Look also for 'mission statements'. There are hundreds if not thousands of agencies out there on the internet (at the time of writing, Google has listings for 1,390,000 for London alone!) and quite often they are run or managed by one person individually. What that website says and the way it is presented may give you a clue to the nature of the person who runs that agency.

Another way to find escort agencies is via women's magazines – the free kind you get on the streets of any major city. Go to the classifieds/general vacancies section. Some people advertise directly for escorts, others use euphemisms. My own inclination is to avoid the ones looking for 'glamour girls' or 'erotic hostesses' – these tend to lead to positions in 'houses' (or brothels), massage parlours, saunas and sleazy clubs. Working in these places is an option, but in my opinion a very bad choice to make: they do not tend to pay well; more often than not you are expected to see well in excess of ten clients a session; and you are more likely to get arrested as quite often they employ a lot of people from abroad, many without legal work papers – consequently Immigration and Vice raid regularly. Look out for straight-talking adverts that say they are looking for escorts. If there is a female contact on the advertisement this is also a good sign.

Now that you've found a few agencies that look promising, it's time to get your mobile phone out. If you haven't got one, get one. You cannot escort without one. You need to be able to make and receive phone calls whenever you are working. It is not just about viable working practices, it is also about safety. While having a phone with you 24/7 ensures that you will be there to receive jobs, it also means that you have a direct line out if anything unpleasant happens. A good reputable agency will require you to ring in and out of a job. This means that when you meet the client and he gives you the agreed fee you phone the agency to let them know you are safe and that the client is happy with you and the set-up. If you are not happy it also means that you can phone your agency to let them know things are not right. Or, in the worst case, phone the police. (In five years of running agencies only one woman I know has ever done this. However, it is always better to be safe than sorry.) You also need to phone the agency when you finish the job or if the client wishes to extend his time with you because the agency will be clocking your time and will be prepared to phone the police should anything happen to you.

If, in a worst-case scenario, you do phone the police, tell them that you met a man and went to his home/hotel. Do not, at this point, tell them that you are an escort. Then tell them what your problem is. Do not be afraid to say after you have told them the problem that you are an escort, it is not illegal to be an escort, but at this point the nature of your call should be the primary concern to the police not what you do for a living. Again, if I was phoning the police on behalf of a woman on a job I would say that my friend had gone wherever it was.

If you already have a mobile it is also a good idea to invest in another that you use just for escorting – a double life in the making! Never use your own landline, Hazel's story explains why:

> I was a very successful escort, but my boyfriend thought I was a freelance clothes designer. Through an agency I started being booked regularly by an American businessman called Paul. At first he visited once a month, then he started sending flowers and cards to me at the agency. Six months later he was crossing the Atlantic at least twice a month to see me! He was bringing me bad lingerie, often buying me dinner and calling himself my American boyfriend. Paul had mistakenly 'fallen

in love' with me. He thought he could 'rescue' me. By this time I was getting thoroughly fed up with him but I made a mistake. One night he phoned my home number. I couldn't believe it, there was Paul on my landline! I didn't remember giving him the number, and then it came to me – I remembered that I had phoned him on it just the once, months before, without withholding the number. My boyfriend was in the room when he phoned as were a couple of my friends. None of them knew what I did for a living – I nearly died! Paul was raving about how much he loved me! God! The man didn't even know who I really was! I pretended it was a wrong number. The next day I phoned the agency to say I would not see him again. But I never felt right about the work again after that. I had to give it up.

Before you use that new mobile to call any agencies decide on a new name and a vague persona. As mentioned in the introduction, most escorts find it easier to have a completely double life. Most friends and lovers will not understand and, unless you are prepared to experiment with losing them or you know what their real feelings on the subject are, it is generally better to create your own escort alter ego. It helps in other ways. A good escort is a good actress. There will be times in an escort's working life when she will have to have sex with someone that she does not find particularly sexually attractive. The best way to deal with this is to think that it is not happening to you, but to your alter ego, eg 'Foxy' the escort. So when 'Foxy' leaves that hotel room with a bag full of money, you can spend it on whatever you need or want. I have in fact met several studying actresses who escorted as part of their research! Your alter ego, if it helps for you to establish her adequately, could wear different clothes than you would normally wear, may speak slightly differently, be a year or two older or younger and may even be sexually different from the person that is you.

However far you take it, start with your name. For instance, I met Suzy, a student nurse, after she replied to an advertisement I'd placed in a women's magazine. She loved sex, was totally broke and had just ended a long relationship. She, like many others, had thought about escorting on and off for quite some time. By the end of our hour-long conversation, I could see Suzy's 'escort persona' and her name was Kelly. She liked it and developed it herself from there.

Now you have decided who your escort alter ego is you can take the next big step. Please bear in mind that at no point are you committed to going any further. You can stop at any time.

How to approach escort agencies

Taking the step to phone your first agency can be somewhat daunting. Do it when you are alone and feeling good about yourself. Many agencies will not discuss terms and conditions with you over the phone – after all they don't know who you are any more than you know who they really are – so they will want to meet you. If a man answers the phone be very wary. Many men start escort agencies as a way of getting to meet girls – unscrupulous and boring, but true! Please bear in mind that the sex industry, particularly in England, has for many years been predominantly run by consistently greedy and exploitative men. If the man wants to meet you at a private place or office ask him if there will be another woman present, if the answer is in the negative ask if you can bring a friend. If he answers in the negative again, hang up. If the agency you have contacted mentions a registration fee, hang up. This is another classic rip-off designed to part you from your money, not make you any! (Many modelling agencies do this too and the same thing applies – if they genuinely want you for a model you should not be required to pay a registration or joining fee.) If anything makes you uncomfortable about your telephone conversation, end it immediately.

If you speak to a man or woman who you instinctively feel all right about on the phone, the next thing to do is to arrange a convenient time and place to meet up. Confirm the date, time and address and arrive on time looking smart/casual. If you have any questions in your mind before you set off to the meeting, write them down. This will help you to decide later on if this is really what you want to do. If you decide at the last moment that this is not what you want to do, phone the agency and cancel.

Getting Started

What You Should Expect From an Agent on First Meeting

At the meeting you should expect to be treated with politeness, honesty and respect. If you feel anything else, leave immediately. You will be asked various things:

- Your names – you will not be asked for your true surname so please don't volunteer it.
- Your age – don't lie unless you *know* you can get away with it, and if you are 18 to 21 and look young take your passport or some other form of identification that confirms you are over 18.
- Your height and measurements; you should also tell them if you have any scars or tattoos – if they want to see your body at this stage, politely decline and leave. If they need to see it, show them your photos or ask them to join you when you arrange your photo shoot (see below).
- Your nationality – again don't lie unless you can get away with it. The amount of illegal Eastern Europeans I have met in London who say they are Italians but have no grasp of the Italian language is astonishing! In most countries if you do not have the legal right to work within that country you should not be escorting.
- Your other work life and consequent availability.
- You will also be asked if you kiss and provide a GFE – this means Girl Friend Experience, that you are happy to kiss, cuddle and be friendly; if you do O/WO – oral sex without a condom; if you do A-Levels – if you do anal

sex; if you are bi – if you are happy having sex with other women; and you may also be asked if you have any BDSM experience – Bondage, Domination and S&M. With these five issues it really is the best policy to be totally honest. If you cannot act well enough to provide a good GFE then you probably should not be escorting; if the thought of O/WO makes you heave then say so; if anal makes you shudder, say so; if you have never been with another girl, be honest. There are no set rules about what you should and should not do. Create your own parameters but the more an agency knows about you and your preferences, what you will and won't do, the more likely they are to book you with suitable clients.

- They will also ask if you have an incall facility – this means that you are prepared to work from your own home or have access to somewhere else where clients can visit you. Don't worry if you haven't; many girls make more than enough just on outcalls – visiting the client at his hotel or residence.

- You will, if the agency works through the internet, be asked about photos. If you have some sexy photos taken by a friend or lover take them along. If you like the agency enough to want to join and don't have any pics, invest in a good photographic session with a reputable photographer. (Yes, there are dodgy photographers out there too! But there are also more female photographers around now who are happy to shoot 'erotic portfolios'.) Do not under any circumstances allow the agency or its representative to trick you into a 'photo package' that you must pay for – it is another classic rip-off ploy. Remember too that the internet is accessed by millions of people daily. If you have a job or are expecting to have a career when you leave university think about blurring the facial features in the pictures you use for escort work. Most agencies will happily do this for you but make sure that you request it from the outset. (If you do find yourself confronted in the future by a colleague or acquaintance that has recognised you on the web my advice is to bluff it out. If it is a man, tell him you are amazed he is the kind of guy using those kinds of sites and you never would have thought it of him. Or say something to the effect of: 'Oh really! Someone who looks like me on something like that! Oh do show me!')

The final thing you will both want to talk about at this meeting is money. There is only one good way for an escort to be paid. That is in cash, by the client, at the beginning of any booking. The escort should then, after completing the job, pay the agency an agreed commission. Commission varies from agency to agency but know what it is before you agree to work with them and decide if what you come out with at the end of a booking after that commission has been deducted is enough to justify what you did to earn it. I personally feel that 20–25 per cent is about right, but many agencies charge over and above this. Do your sums and work out what you will end up with in your hand at the end of the day. Only you can decide how much your time and body is worth, but never undervalue yourself.

What You Should Not Expect from Agencies on First Meeting

Primarily, as I have already stated, you should not be expected to pay any kind of registration fee or money up front to join an agency. If an agency suggests a photographer to you for your escort shots ask to see a portfolio of his work and compare his charges to other similar practitioners in the field. You should not have to pay for your web page on an escort agency's site. If they want to put you up on their website, the cost of adding an extra page is, believe me, minimal. You should not have to pay all of your first job's fee to the agency as a joining cost. Be wary, it has been brought to my attention that agencies do this without telling you till you are about to do your first job with them.

The second major thing to watch out for when meeting a new agency is the casting couch syndrome. Too many women to mention have fallen foul of this manipulative male practice. The line: 'How do I know you can suck my clients' cocks if you won't suck mine?' should have you heading straight for the door. Similarly, if a male agent wants to see you naked or topless without another woman there – bye, bye. It comes back to self-respect – if the agent is prepared to pay you an agreed fee for you to perform fellatio on him and you are happy to do it then that is fine, otherwise know that he is a time-wasting self-obsessed loser who can't get women any other way and who will probably rip you off at some point if you do go to work for him.

Getting Started

Meg is an American graduate who was travelling the world on a budget after completing her degree:

> I met Alex through a woman I met at a party. She said he was a good guy who ran a reputable escort agency and if I were struggling he would help me out till I got myself sorted. We arranged to meet in a nice apartment in a red light district. He seemed quite personable. I told him I had never done anything like this before. He told me that usually he checked out all the girls he hired before recommending them to clients. I had sex with him. I hated it and him. He was kind of slimy. He got me a bit of work and sometimes he let me stay at his apartment when I had nowhere else to go but I always had to have sex with him in exchange.

Meg's story is quite common. When I met her she seemed somewhat downtrodden and eventually she gave up sex work and returned home.

You should not expect, nor should you agree, to being paid by cheque after the event. Another common rip-off is the agency that says it collects money from its 'membership' on a regular basis and can only pay you by cheque two weeks after you do a job. Although there are various 'men's sex clubs' out there whose members contribute regularly to a central pot, if you are hired by one of them you should always be paid up front and in cash for anything you do.

Your First Job

You have met an agency you like and they have put you up on their website. You have let them know your availability and you are waiting for that first call. Don't panic but do be prepared. Keep a small, discreet bag of clothes and make-up ready. If you have opted for discretion and not telling family and friends, a nice white lie I have found useful in the past is that you are doing freelance promotions work. The kind where you have to look a bit glamorous, stroll around bars and clubs, have fun and give away things like free cigarettes, lighters and obnoxious new alcopops. This easily explains why you get calls at odd times of the day and night and why you need to look good for 'the job'. Just smile and bluff.

The first call comes. The agency will provide you with details of the client's name, address, telephone number and sometimes his required preferences. Any reputable agency will have run a security check on the client by taking the client's name and accommodation details and checking them with Directory Enquiries or the hotel in question (this will be explained in full in Chapter Seven). The agency does not generally discuss your services or your fee with the client. The agency merely facilitates the introduction. Whatever happens between you and the client is legally just between two consenting adults. We all know that we are selling sex here but the agency cannot outwardly state it because they are not legally selling sex, they are merely facilitating one person spending a pre-booked amount of time with another person.

Getting Started

You telephone the client, withholding your number always. Now is the time for your instinct to really come into play. This is your first contact with a person you are potentially going to become intimate with. Use your escort alter ego to sell yourself to him over the phone while listening out very carefully for any sign from him that you will not get along. Be businesslike and intelligent but sensual.

Arrange a realistic time to meet the client – do not tell him that you can be there in half an hour when you are on the other side of town without cab fare, though if he is desperate you can always suggest that he pays for your taxi when you get there. If he is in a hotel ask him where in the hotel his room is situated. Find out what he would like you to wear and be honest with him if you can't manage it because you are miles from home and you haven't got your suspender belt and stockings with you. Find out if there is any particular service he would like from you and be honest with him about whether you will be happy to provide it. If it has not already come up now is the time to talk about money. Whatever your agreed fee with the agency is, stick to it. Do not try to charge more, do not ever charge less unless the client is prepared to negotiate extra time in which case a small discount for a third hour is reasonable and allows the client to think he is getting a 'deal'. You then telephone your agency back advising them of the time, length and agreed fee for the booking.

As discussed above, any reputable agency will clock watch on your behalf. If you know you are going to be late for a booking, telephone the client and then telephone the agency to let them know how late you are running. When you get to the job get the agreed fee from your client and telephone the agency to let them know you are safe and that everything is fine – ie that you have the money and you are alright with the client. If, at any point during your inter-action with him – from initial telephone call to him opening the door to you – anything at all says to you 'No! This is not right!' or 'This is wrong!' then get out. This is always a choice. Your choice. Even if this happens after you have taken the money from him – simply give it back to him, apologise and leave.

Now you are down to the reality of escorting – interacting with the client. Ideally he will have discussed his require-ments with you on the telephone so you will have an idea of what his sexual reality is. When you are with him try to get to know him: behave like a girlfriend, chat, kiss, cuddle, shower together. These activities have two functions. One is that you get to know the person you are interacting with a little. The other is that the more varied you make the time the more fun it will be for the both of you. Depending on who you are with, an hour can go by in the flash of an eye or can seem to drag on forever – the more you put into it sexually and intellectually the more you are likely to get out of it.

Learn from your clients, as Mya did:

I was working in a 'house' in Queensland, Australia.
It was only my second job ever. I gave the guy what
I thought was a reasonably passable blowjob.

After he came I asked him if he had enjoyed it and he told me that he'd had better. I was a bit taken aback and a little hurt to be honest. But I thought, learn from this experience! I asked him to show me how he liked it best. I've never had a complaint since!

When the agreed time is up leave politely, unless he would like to pay for some more of your time of course, and telephone the agency to let them know you are safe. Treat yourself to a cab home. Most clients are genuinely okay people who will quite often pay for your cab home, but do not expect it.

There is, in all of this, one factor we cannot do without in the equation – The Client.

Chapter Two

Clients

Like any industry, sex work would not exist without its customers: clients, punters, johns, users. (While the term 'user' may seem strange, we use this word because many men deal with escorts as if they, or the commodity they sell, that is sex, were in fact a drug. They are quite literally addicted to the purchasing of sex.) Call them what you will, there would be no escorting and no prostitution without the primary factor of men and their money. While men are prepared to pay for sexual favours there will always be prostitution.

Many men never use escorts. The concept of paying for sex never occurs to them. They can be sympathetic, like John:

> I went to Thailand and in a bar I met these girls. We were backpacking and obviously didn't look like serious punters. We got talking. Their whole thing was that they were working to support their

families so why would they work in a bar for 18 hours a day for 1,000 baht a day when they could shag a tourist for 10,000 baht an hour. They were nice girls and I wanted for them to be able to change but they maintained it was okay for them because it was for their families.

Some men use hookers once in their life, quite often as a drunken dare, and feel guilty about it for the rest of their lives. Other men, however, become serial escort clients. They get off on paying for beauty, intelligence, youth, companionship and some kind of sexual fulfilment.

Other men perceive women who work in the sex industry as dirty, diseased and unworthy of respect. As Andrew says:

I wouldn't buy a whore a drink, let alone pay her for sex.

Please don't make the assumption that all men or all clients are the same. Like any societal sub-group made up of individuals they all vary. Non-clients tend to be divided in the way that Andrew and John are – one group despising the fact of sex work and the women who do it; the other feeling a sort of 'social worker sympathy' for sex workers. The same applies to users or clients. Some men who use escorts despise themselves for doing so, and consequently the women they hire become the objects of their disgust. On the other hand some clients adore the women, and the process and the buzz of a sexual interaction in which they feel they have total control because they are paying for it.

Some men will admit to using an escort once, like Jacques:

> I was drunk; I did it for the crack. It wasn't particularly satisfying. Like going shopping. Which I do not enjoy either.

Escort clients are old, young, ugly, handsome, fat, thin, stupid and intelligent. Just like the rest of us they are multi-faceted. Their motivations vary but what you have to remember is that punters or clients are people. They have lives, needs and jobs, just like you.

Generally, the amount of the cash transaction equates to the quality of the client. So, if you are selling your body in a cheap brothel or on the streets for a small amount of money the chances are that the 'clients' you will attract will be the disaffected, the drunk, the physically challenged, the dodgy and the poor. As Sarah attests:

> I had been an escort and glamour model for two years when I had a bit of bad luck and found myself in a really bad financial situation. I went to work in a working flat, a brothel. Twelve hour shifts with a client every half hour. The rates were on a sliding scale depending on what the punter wanted – £20 for a hand job, £30 for a blowjob and £40 for full sex. 10 per cent went to the maid, 40 per

cent to the house and I got 50 per cent. It was awful. These men were the lowest level of society – mostly drunk, barely literate and quite often with something physically wrong with them. Because the place was so cheap you could end up doing eight hours of your shift hardly seeing anyone but the minute the pubs closed the place would be packed, the Madame running around stressing all the girls to 'do' the punters as fast as possible. The sheets didn't get changed, there was no security if a punter got nasty and it was the lowest point in my working life.

Sarah's story exemplifies almost the lowest level at which one can function in the sex industry. I do not recommend working at this level whatever your financial reality. It does not have to be that grim. Which is not to say that you will not find the traits described above in men who will pay hundreds of pounds or dollars for an hour or more of your sexual favours. However the chances are that they will be cleaner, more respectful and the environment in which you do it will be nicer.

The demands and reasons for women and companionship as well as sex by men are manifold. Again, try to remember that clients are people just like you. In my experience, if treated with respect 90 per cent of escort clients will do the same in return. Also bear in mind that clients can become friends. But do not confuse the issue – if a client becomes a friend that does not entitle him to free sex. Remember your body is your income. But be open-minded to all opportunities, as Maria is:

> The rules are quite simple. Never talk about your private life and do not disclose too much personal information about yourself. We all do, to a greater or lesser extent, but you are always aware and guarded about what you say for the most part – after all, you don't know who this person is. Instinct does a very good job of keeping you in check most of the time but there will be the occasional client you meet where, somehow, you just don't feel the need to pretend, on any level. You really 'click'. The few times this has happened to me with clients have been wonderful and I now have one very established friendship, which I cherish, and another beautiful friendship in its infancy.
>
> 'Harry' was the first client who I became friends with and we both agreed, on the same day, coincidently, that we should terminate our 'business arrangement' and carry on seeing each other on a friends-only basis. This move worked well for both of us because as our friendship has blossomed, the whole process of being paid/paying for sex just didn't feel right anymore.
>
> The notion that clients and escorts can genuinely become friends seems alien to many. I've had a few raised eyebrows myself when mentioning my 'ex-client, now friend' relationships. 'How

can that be?!' people ask. Most people's idea is that all clients are really hated deep down by the 'victim' sex worker. This is false. At the end of the day people meet some of their friends at work. Period. Receptionists make friends with office workers. Barmen make friends with waiters; similarly escorts make friends with clients. And good friends they can make too! It is not perhaps the most usual way to meet someone but I think it can produce some incredibly deep connections; after all, you have been with that person intimately and may know more about them already than all their other friends may know in a lifetime.

Most men are driven to pay for sex by fairly simple reasons or urges: the wife or partner who won't or can't be bothered to fulfil sexual requests or needs; the frequent business traveller; the disabled; the celebrator; the virgin; the fetishist; the escort addict; the simply lonely; and finally, the worst of all, the misogynist psycho.

The Client Whose Wife/Partner Won't Do What he Wants Sexually

Many men share their lives with women whom they love but with whom they cannot be sexually honest. Whether it be something as simple as a desire to have an interaction with a woman in sexy lingerie who will suck his cock to completion or an overwhelming need to have a threesome. If his wife or partner is not approachable the simple thing to do is to hire someone to fulfil those needs for him. Someone who isn't going to tell his wife, who is going to give him the exact gratification he requires and who is not going to turn into a blackmailing bunny boiler overnight. As Tim says:

> As an upper-middle-class Jewish lawyer from a good family I married an upper-middle-class Jewish woman from another equally good family. I love her; she is a good wife and mother. But I was in torment for the first five years of our marriage. We've never really talked about sex and did not have sex before we married; we just do it with the lights out. I like a woman who will dress up in stockings and suspenders and high heels that will let me worship her legs with the lights on before she gives me a blow job to completion. I think my wife would have a heart attack before asking for a divorce if I mentioned any of this to her. I go to see Kathy at her centrally located apartment, 15 minutes walk from my office, once a month. No one knows but she and I, it's safe and totally distanced from my 'real' life. I get what I need and no one is hurt or any the wiser.

The Frequent Business Traveller

Due to the ever-diminishing size of our world many men who work in international banking, IT, politics and multi-national corporations quite often find themselves in a different city every other week. More often than not they have more than one home in more than one city. These men are hard-working, high-flying executives whose primary motivation in life is their careers and money. The best way for men in these positions to relax and get their sexual fulfilment is to hire an escort. They do not have the time to trawl around bars chatting up girls who at the end of the night may not even 'put out'. All they have to do is access the internet, find the appropriate location, pick the woman they would like to see, make a phone call and – hey presto! – within the hour they have what they want, where they want it and they will happily pay for it because mutually beneficial commercial transactions are how they deal with the rest of their working existence. As Steve says:

> I spend my life between London, New York, Los Angeles, Milan, Paris and Berlin. Some weeks I am on a plane every other day. I have a girlfriend at home but because of both our work commitments we can sometimes go a whole month without seeing each other. Most days I work 12–14 hours and at the end of the day the last thing I want to do is to sit in a soulless hotel room on my own. I love my girlfriend but she won't go with other girls and she won't do anal. So, if I feel like having something like that I just call one of my favourite agencies where ever I am. They know what I like – beautiful, tall, slender women who do CIM [cum in mouth]

and anal, they send her over and we have some fun. I spend on average 1,000–2,000 euros per month. I did try stopping but I just do not have the time for the frustration of trying to find a casual sexual partner without commitment.

The Marginalised

Physically disabled people are quite often minimised by society on many levels, their sexuality being one of the least recognised human conditions by the able-bodied. Because a lot of women in the sex industry feel themselves marginalised from society in general, many, though not all, have a much more open view with regard to 'body politics' and can enhance the lives of disabled men who society not only sees as legless but also sexless. Richard's story is typical:

> I was the CEO of a big company before my accident four years ago. I am paralysed from the neck down, apart from, ironically, my penis, which works fine, though I cannot touch it myself. My mental acuity is, if anything, sharper than before my accident. I was married and though my wife tried hard she could not get to grips with looking after or having sex with someone who could not move. I started using escorts who I have found to be sensitive, caring, affectionate and above all non-judgemental about my condition.

Clients

It is not just the disabled who come into this category, however, as Regina shows us:

> I work with a lot of obese and overly-obese clients as they find it difficult to meet anyone to have a sexual encounter with (I think they got hold of me by word-of-mouth). Most of them find girls very intimidating or/and have very low self-esteem level.

The Celebrator

Like the one-off escort client who did it because he got drunk another type of client is what I call 'The Celebrant'. He is the guy who has just made that first big deal or million at work, the guy who just won 10,000 in a casino or the guy, after a successful business lunch, that wants to impress his friends or colleagues. It would seem that the way to celebrate is to buy a load of cocaine, book a large room at your nearest Hilton and hire a couple of escort girls. It is very easy for an escort to get caught up in drug use and abuse, particularly with a celebrating client, but I do not advise doing drugs with clients if you can help it, as it can seriously impair your judgement – the same thing applies to excessive alcohol use. Kirstie's story highlights the excesses that people can go to.

> I got a job with another girl in the Hilton. It was two guys who had been drinking and doing coke for their business lunch. By the time we got there at about ten o'clock they were really trashed. We

drank champagne and took coke with them and talked for ages. Earlier one of them had just won a load of money playing roulette and he was planning to blow it all that night. He had booked this enormous suite and had already bought copious amounts of drugs. He took a liking to me so I went with him when we decided to go into the bedroom. He wanted me to stay the night and bring my girlfriend over too.

Melinda, my girlfriend, is gay and only does lesbian shows. But this client had had so much cocaine that I knew there would be very little sex and that both my girlfriend and the client would be fine. I also invited Chloe, an escort who I thought these guys would like. She is the Barbie doll fantasy escort – not very bright with fake boobs, hair, teeth and so on. The three of us basically performed threesomes and foreplay for a few hours as well as rinsing their coke.

I didn't like this guy – he had not called his wife to say he wasn't coming home (come on, I am a lesbian and bragging about that stuff pisses me off), he was also rude, arrogant and demanding. I was so broke and I was so trashed at that point that I just didn't care. Coke on escort jobs is often limitless – everyone involved is playing roles, you're in a hotel and it is all not real, so the coke also becomes unreal and you just end up taking so much. I think sometimes the clients are on an

Clients

almost self-destructive path – past enjoyment into the point of being so trashed that they are not aware that they have a wife and a job to go to the following day. Anyway then the client's friend suddenly freaks out – it's all got too blurry for him. He wants to go home so he gets dressed but he can't find his sock. The night then turns into the mission of finding his sock. But we are all really out of it and no one but him really cares or knows how to look for things. So for over an hour we are looking, but because we are trashed in really silly places like under ashtrays. We never found the sock and he went home with out it. After he left the remaining client decided to buy some Ketamin. He had never had it before but wanted something to take the edge off the coke. He had a tiny line and he liked it – he found it relaxing. But then somebody – probably Chloe – thought it would be funny if he had a huge line and he went into a complete state of Ketamin madness and my girlfriend and Chloe decided they'd had enough and wanted to leave. The client didn't want me to go, so I had to stay and look after him. He was so freaked out. I had to put him in the bath, get him drinking orange juice to bring him down and reassure him that he would be okay for his meeting – he had a presentation at nine. I don't know if he was – I felt wrecked and fuzzy at midday and that was after sleeping so I am guessing that he called in sick.

In Good Company

Be very wary of clients who use drugs. Cocaine particularly can have a very unpredictable effect on people. Do not purchase drugs on behalf of a client, it will put you deeply into the realms of behaving illegally.

The Virgin

Unfortunately some men have trouble entering the sexual arena. Whether it be fear of failure or fear of ridicule, the virgin is quite often better off 'losing his cherry' to a woman who is going to treat him with respect, who is not going to laugh at him and who will potentially teach him how to treat other women well for the rest of his life. Sometimes a father figure or older male role model will facilitate this and sometimes the young man himself will find that his inability to talk to non-virginal women, his general embarrassment and ignorance will force him to what he can see is his only course of action if he is ever going to lose his virginal millstone. As Stuart's story shows:

> I was 23 before I lost my virginity. To an escort. Women always said I was not bad looking, they also said I was a nice guy. But none of them wanted to have sex with me. It got to the point where I could think about nothing else. All my mates lost theirs when we were in our teens and I was beginning to feel like some kind of freak. I was masturbating over magazines, the internet, my own imagination, anything — it was getting out of hand! Then I found Teri on the web. She was perfect

– blonde, beautiful, perfectly proportioned and intelligent. I made an appointment and went to see her. It was the best thing that could have happened to me. She took things slowly, didn't laugh at me when I came too quickly – several times – and showed me how to make her come. I no longer see her for sex but we did become friends. And the women I have been with since think I am a fantastic lover. Thanks to Teri.

The Fetishist

The fetishist is the individual whose sexual requirements are considered to be so far out there that he cannot even bring himself to mention them to women in general. The guy who likes to be urinated or shat on; the guy who likes to spank or be spanked or even just a simple bit of BDSM with sex. A good escort should not be phased by any sexual peccadillo but should take it in her stride and either decline politely or get on with the requested act, as Sandra has done quite often. These two stories of Sandra's represent the extremes:

Our flat was a big hang-out for gay men. Druggies, clubbers and rent boys were always coming to stay. At one point we had a boy called John living with us. He was a big time rent boy with a bad drug problem – he would do anything for money. One of his clients was a man with a fetish for being faeciated on – the more the better. This man was not what you would expect at all. He was a businessman with a wife and 2.4 children. But the people who are most normal in life always seem to have the most out there fetishes and fantasies. Faeciation is actually quite common. Sex is often if not always about power – the taking, receiving and giving of it. Being faeciated on is the ultimate humiliation, leaving you powerless. It is usually popular with people who are in powerful jobs – a kind of expensive and unhygienic form of escapism. But this client of John's was the biggest fan I ever met. He preferred boys but would settle for girls, including myself, and once a week he would come round to our flat and lie in our bath. John and whoever he could recruit would queue outside and we would go in one at a time or occasionally in pairs. And have a shit on him. He liked it anywhere including in his mouth so that he could eat it. I think the most was six people. There were always arguments among us over who went last because as you can imagine the smell just worsened as each person went in. All of us referred to him as Mr Shit. We would be given 24 hours' notice and would eat loads of fibre and not go to the toilet so we were 'full' for him, after we had done our part he always masturbated and cleaned up all the mess, put on his suit and gave us £80–£100 per person. Whenever my friends asked why I did something like that I would just say, 'Well my toilet isn't going to pay me is it?'

Clients

(I do not recommend living or working with drug users.)

I have a client who has very particular tastes – the girl's arse has to be perfect for one thing, he likes them small and pert. He like escorts to be wild and 'up for it' and he likes bisexuals and threesomes. And he is very into rubber. He will often take the girls to Ann Summers first – as long as they don't charge him for that time – and buy them rubber or latex knickers and suspenders. He even provides talcum powder to get the latex stockings on, and let me tell you they are the most unsexy, unflattering and difficult things to put on – you have to jump and wobble and bend and twist while you pull them tightly on, they are filled with talc which by the time you have both legs pulled up is all over the floor. I have occasionally met this guy already wearing the stockings and nothing else but my coat, just because putting them on in the room kind of kills it. Once you are dressed he likes to play around. He is into foreplay and doggy style but you have to also keep drinking water because before he comes he likes to place a towel on the floor, lie down and have you piss in his mouth and on his chest. You have to control, stagger and direct your piss to his instruction. It's difficult until you get the hang of it but once you know how to do it, it can give you a power rush. If there are two girls, he really likes it if one of you takes his mouth and one his genitals and you try to time it together. He also loves to swap stories. He has lots of dirty stories from around the world and every time we meet we discuss our latest sex adventures. Clients often like to hear what you get up to on other jobs – before I had enough to get me through an overnight booking I would just make them up.

The Escort Addict

This is the man who can *only* have sex with escorts. In his home city he will have investigated every prostitute within his price range that fits in with his physical and sexual requirements. Sometimes he will see the same girl over and over again. Sometimes he will see a different girl every time. For an agency these clients are gold dust. They never go away. Even as they get older they keep going. It is almost like they are driven, only death or exposure stops them. These are the men who live on the internet review sites (more of them later in this chapter) who compare notes and 'chat' with other clients. They are the bread and butter of the escort industry. The turn-on for them is partially the sex but it is also the transaction that is taking place that gets them going.

The Lonely

The lonely, too, are a large proportion of our clientele. These are the men who are divorced or widowed or the men who have never been able to get on well with women sexually because of shyness. Divorce can make a man feel

Clients

like he will never trust a woman again – particularly if he believes that he was the injured party, and if he is paying support or alimony to the woman who he feels has ruined his life. Hiring an escort can change that perspective, as Paul found out:

My wife decided that I wasn't capable of understanding her any more, whatever that means! She found a man who apparently did understand her. She ruined my business in the divorce courts and I can only see my kids once a month. I never wanted to see another woman again let alone have sex with one. Then one night alone in my apartment I couldn't stop thinking about sex so I phoned an agency and got Heidi. She was a tonic. When she arrived I was a bit nervous, never having done this sort of thing before. I offered her a drink and we sat down. Before we had finished the bottle of wine I had told her my entire story of woe and she was just so sympathetic. She was very sensitive and understanding. We talked for the whole of the hour and then she explained that she could only stay if I could pay her for another hour. I got angry then till she calmed me down. Heidi was merely performing an agreed business transaction; she wasn't being like my ex-wife and trying to squeeze me dry financially. Heidi said she liked me and that she would be happy to come back the next night and would ask the agency if I could have a discount on a two-hour booking. Not bad considering I had spent an hour with this gorgeous girl whining about my sorry life. I booked her the next evening and we had a great time – the best sex ever. Now I only have sex with escorts.

Men who have lost wives or lovers to death can also benefit from using an escort. One of the most isolating things about close personal bereavement is the lack of touch. An escort can be the much-needed therapy that a recently bereaved man needs, as Grace explains:

I met Mark when he called me about six months after his wife died. I went to see him at his home. The poor man had barely left the place since her death. It seemed quite obvious to me that he did not want sex with me. We chatted for a while and I just stroked his hand. When he started to get a bit tearful I offered to give him a massage. He loved it. He said I made him feel connected to the world again. I saw him for about three months – we never had sex, we just chatted a bit, mostly about his life with his wife and I would give him a good warm loving rubdown.

The Misogynist/Psycho

Finally, last, but by no means the least prevalent, is the psycho. He is the nightmare client. He is the verbal or physical abuser, the guy that pays who then either tries to rip you off afterwards or feels that the exchange of money for sex means that he owns you in entirety. He is the guy that will dive into your handbag while you are in the toilet (so take it with you!); he is the guy with a pile of twenties, but the only real one is the one on the top, the rest being counterfeit (always check your money properly!); he is 'The Big Spender' whose cash card isn't working for some strange reason (always remember: no cash up front – no sexual interaction! Becky's story below highlights this); he is the man that will try to persuade you to have sex without a condom (there are a surprising number of men who want to have unprotected sex with sex workers – they will try to persuade you that they have been tested but the sheer stupidity of this request is obvious. Never have unprotected sex. *Ever!*).

Becky's story is by no means unique:

> I received a phone call one day from a woman who said she ran an agency and that she had got my number from the webmaster of one of the agencies I am listed with – this seemed strange but I ignored it. She said she had a very wealthy client who had seen my pictures on the internet and wanted to see me, but he would only deal through her. Stupidly, ignoring all the rules, I arranged to meet him. I met up with KJ on the following Thursday night. He had a gorgeous car with a driver, £4,000 and three grams of cocaine. He was very arrogant and boasted about the interior

design jobs he had done, the celebrities he knew, the apartments he owned and how much money and influence he had. As a lover KJ was . . . cruel but manageable. I spent six hours with him which he paid me for and we agreed to meet the following Sunday for me to spend the whole night with him at his house outside of the city. On the Sunday I duly made my way there and KJ didn't have any cash on him so we went out to get some. His ATM card, he said, wasn't working properly and he asked if he could pay me in the morning. Because he had thrown so much cash around on our previous meeting I thought it would be okay. I had arrived at 7 pm. I stayed with him till 5 am the following morning when he threw me out of his house screaming abuse at me. He called me a filthy whore, said I had just been with him for the money. I mean, why else would I be there? And he left me miles from the centre of the city where I live without even enough money for the train fare home. As soon as I got home I let other women I knew in the industry know what had happened because he had boasted to me about how many escorts he hired per month. It turned out that he had been perpetrating this kind of stunt on a regular basis and that at least four other women had been victims of exactly the same kind of trick within the previous six months.

Clients

Men like these should be heavily discouraged, immediately reported to the police and/or other working women, whichever is appropriate, and posted up on the appropriate sites on the internet like Escort Watch and Punter Net.

Sugar Daddies

For most 'career escorts' the ideal is to find the one client who will keep you in the style to which you wish to be accustomed for life. Ideally he will buy you an apartment and pay you a monthly sum in order for you not to share your sexual favours with anyone else. Or you may fall in love with each other. This may sound like a dream but it does happen. It is, however, very rare. Tricia was a networks systems analyst with expensive tastes who escorted occasionally to supplement her income. She says:

> I met Danny through another client of mine. After I had seen him two or three times it became obvious that it was more than just the normal client and escort relationship. The sex was amazing; we enjoyed each other's company, had a laugh and liked a lot of the same things in life. Within two months we had agreed that if he paid an agreed amount into my bank account every month I would not see anyone else. We fell in love. We carried on like that for a year. Last year we got married and now we live in the Caribbean. I could not be happier.

In Good Company

Tricia's story is unusual. It is the fairy tale with the happy ending for 'The Scarlet Woman'. Do not expect this from every client. Although love does occur in the strangest of places, clients as a rule are not looking for it, they are looking for a commercial/sexual transaction without emotional commitment. But keep your eyes and your mind open to all opportunities that come your way from any direction.

Clients and the Internet

Due to the burgeoning nature of the escorting industry over the last five to eight years, coupled with an internet technology almost anyone can easily access, the web has become the largest forum for people to buy and sell sex. Consequently, among clients there has become an almost club-like atmosphere on the internet. Men join sites like www.Captain69.co.uk, www.punterlink.co.uk and RAPS (at www.aspd.net) where they can write reviews, compare notes and quite often stroke their own and each other's egos over their real or imagined sexual prowess. These sites have both a positive and negative affect for the sex worker. If you get a good review you are sorted for work for the life of your career. Men believe each other. If one man on an appropriate platform says Girl A is a great fuck, gives the best blow job he ever had and does anal then any other men accessing that platform will be checking that girl out within minutes. Her phone will go red hot and the work will pile in. On the other hand, get a bad review and you may never work again.

Clients

> Katrina was an Austrian design student supple-
> menting her course with sex work. She had very
> slightly protruding teeth but otherwise was blonde,
> blue-eyed, petite and sexy. She saw a client who
> posted a review within 48 hours of seeing her. The
> essence of which was that: 'while it was a pretty lit-
> tle thing, its teeth were so bad you would not want
> to kiss it'. Katrina never got a job again.

You can, of course, just change your name and photographs if this happens to you, but please be aware that a lot of these people are not all as gullible as some of them may seem.

Though these forums have less individual impact as more of them come into being on the internet, the two main points here are: 1) if you have a regular client who you get on well with do not hesitate to ask him to write a review of you. It will give him a buzz and it will do your business the world of good. And 2) be very nice to all clients because you do not know what will happen after you leave them.

Non-Clients

We cannot finish this chapter without talking about the 'non-clients'. I call them left-handed mouse users (work it out for yourself!), time-wasters, wankers or tossers. These are the guys who ring on withheld phone numbers, breathe and hang up. The men with impeccable accents and voices who will talk for too long on the phone and will be getting off then and there. Or the men who will make a booking with you, then not show up without even doing you the courtesy of cancelling. There is very little we can do about these men except keep their names, phone numbers and modus operandi on file. If every escort and agency did this and put it into a central database there would be meltdown!

* * *

Every individual has different tastes. Men are not just attracted to tall, young, thin blondes with big breasts. Just as woman do not just fancy big, handsome 'Marlboro men' with huge cocks. Thousands of men every day all over the world pay for sex. Their tastes and desires are as varied as humanity. Clients are, quite often, in their own minds, sexual heroes. They pay you for confirmation of this. Your success as an escort is in your ability to stroke ego as well as you stroke cock.

Chapter Three

The Reality of Escorting

On a day-to-day basis it can be quite easy to incorporate escorting into your 'normal' existence. If you are organised and logical then you and your escort alter ego can live quite happily side-by-side. Know that the ultimate reality in all of this is sex. Out of 1,000 escorting jobs, 999 mean sex. Know what you will and won't do. Be honest about it and stick to your guns. Do not let anyone coerce or force you into doing anything you do not want to do. Whatever else you do, know your job, learn your craft and be the best at what you do.

The Importance of Communication

Although good communication seems obvious it cannot be stressed how important it is for both your success and your safety. We are lucky enough to live in a time where technology allows us to be contactable and to contact others 24/7. Use this technology to your advantage. Never switch your phone off. It is your line to work. It is your line to help should anything ever go wrong. It may save your life.

As discussed in Chapter One, you will be expected to ring the client. Do so as soon as you get the call from your agency. Do not leave it for 15 minutes. It is possible that he will be looking at many more escorts than you on the internet and will choose the one that gets back to him the quickest. Just because a client requests you personally does not mean that you do not have competition – the internet has thousands of women selling themselves, remember that you are just one of them.

When speaking with clients on the phone always withhold your number (remember Hazel's story from Chapter One, page 25). In England just dial 141 before you dial the client's number, in America dial *67 and in Australia it is 1831. Always keep your phone safe and with you at all times. If you lose your phone let your agent know as soon as possible – some agents do worry when they cannot get hold of a girl. As previously stated, always phone in and out of jobs and always let your agency know when you are not available.

Bearing that in mind, when you actually speak to the client on the phone understand that you are selling yourself. Just like in a job interview the impression you make in that first 30 seconds of communication is vital. Be sexy, be seductive, but above all be honest. Do not tell a client that you are happy to do things that you are not. It is better to be honest and lose a booking than it is to find yourself in the position of having to deal with expectations you are not prepared or able to fulfil.

The Reality of Escorting

Once you have phoned the client call your agency immediately to tell them the outcome of your phone conversation. This will let them know not to double-book you and keep them informed of the timing you have agreed with your client. If you are running late for your booking always phone the client and the agency to keep them informed of your progress. This is a courtesy to both your client, who is expecting you, and your agency, who may be worrying about you. When you get to the job and have got your cash upfront, phone the agency to let them know that you are fine and that you have the agreed amount of cash for the time booked. If the booking is for an hour, call the agency at the end of that hour to let them know you are safe and either about to leave the job or have left. If you phone on the hour and are still with your client always phone the agency again after you leave his home or hotel. This is a safety precaution. It lets the agency know that you are in fact safe and heading on your own way. If your client is having so much fun with you (and he has the cash) that he would like to extend your time together, phone the agency to let them know that you will be with your client for another hour or half. Agencies are not psychic. Nothing is more likely to get you taken off an agency's books than a predilection for drinking too much with your client and forgetting to phone in. An agent's perspective:

> I was running someone else's agency and they had a very successful escort called Maggie. She was vibrant, busty and very popular. However she

drank to excess, used cocaine and regularly failed to call in and out of jobs. She was a nightmare because I never knew whether she was safe or not. In the end I wanted to fire her but because she was such a high earner the agency owner would not let me – he could not have cared less about the woman involved but only saw her as a cash cow. Eventually I just stopped giving her work because she could not understand why this was an issue. If something really bad had happened to her I could not have lived with it. The responsibility we take is too high to risk on someone who is consistently flaky. I stopped working for that agency about a month later.

If your agency is particularly scrupulous, neglecting to keep them informed might find you in the embarrassing position of having the police knock at your client's hotel door.

Finally, most agencies do not mind when you work as long as they know. Do not tell an agency you are available and then switch your phone off. If you have said you are available and then change your mind or something else comes up just call or text to let them know. Nothing is more annoying for an agent than to spend their time 'selling' an escort to a client only to discover that they cannot get hold of that escort. The bottom line is: Keep your lines of communication open at all times. It will get you work and keep you safe.

The Reality of Escorting

Preparation

Travelling to jobs and arriving in the right state physically and mentally is an important thing to learn. If you are leading a double life and not devoting yourself to escorting 24/7 then you will need to keep your escort alter ego in your bag. Ideally in a bag of her own. This should contain:

- condoms;
- lubricant;
- make-up;
- stockings and suspenders;
- a change of knickers;
- sea sponges if you are menstruating – these are always good to carry with you for a multitude of purposes but primarily, unless you are an extremely heavy bleeder, they enable you to work every day of the year if you choose;
- a street map of your city;
- enough cash for a taxi ride;
- your mobile phone charger;
- and, most importantly, paper and pen to write the details of jobs down with.

If you are meeting the client at his home or hotel, without several hours notice, and you are out and about when you get the call without your 'bag of whore tricks', then be honest with him. Tell him you are wearing jeans and that you only have the basest of make-up on. This is the only fair thing to do because the client is generally interested in you based on what he has seen of you on the internet, where we have to assume you got yourself looking sexed-up and gorgeous for your photo shoot. In my experience most clients do not mind if they are forewarned. Most clients also know that if they have a specific requirement in mind that they are far more likely to get it if they give a few hours notice. As Scott says:

> I know what I want and I know what I like – two young and genuinely bisexual girls with a large selection of toys. I know, from experience, that organising this for 9 pm on a Friday night in a big city at 8 pm is futile. I always call the agency of my choice at least three to four days beforehand.

Scott is an unusual but very sensible regular client. He generally gets exactly what he wants when he wants it.

Hotel bookings can be a lot of fun though they are fraught with exposure possibilities. Consequently there are some very logical guidelines to follow. When speaking to a client who is booked into a hotel that you are not familiar with, ask him where his floor and room are in relation to reception. When you get to the hotel go straight to the room as per his directions. When you walk through the hotel lobby be dressed smart/casual. Look like a business-woman, do not dress like a tart. If the client wants you to look 'slutty' take the outfit with you. Carry your things in a briefcase. Be confident. Nothing will get you thrown out of a major hotel in any city quicker than looking cheap and lost in an expensive hotel foyer.

The Reality of Escorting

The Job Itself

Now we come down to the 'meat' of what being an escort is all about. Sex. Be under no illusions. The job itself is about sex. You don't have to like sex to be a good escort but it helps. This is a breakdown of an hour with a client. You meet at the pre-arranged time and place. You get your fee and phone your agency. You are providing a 'GFE' – a true 'girl-friend experience'. He wants you to treat him like a man you really fancy, a man you really want (in my experience most clients think they are more handsome and more sexy than they actually are in real life – it's called narcissism). Fiona who was a sex worker for seven years gives this advice:

> **Take care of your clients**. Make them feel how they want to feel. Two things most men want is to feel sexy, and to feel powerful. If you want them to be regulars it is your job to make them feel this way, even the men who are as appealing as a ten mile run after a Saturday night on the town. You know what I mean when I say a man's 'got it' or he has not 'got it', well most 'have it' . . . play along. Give them the best they've ever had. To succeed in this business you need regular clients, to get regular clients you need to give them what they don't get from any where else, when they meet you it is your task to make them never want to leave. If you can achieve this they will be planning their return visit before they have even left.

In Good Company

The power of three. During each meeting you need to make three separate compliments that are believable, each comment needs to be within the boundaries of reality so don't go telling a great big fat client that he looks athletic, tell him he looks powerful and protective. So why *three*? If you say more than three it sounds too much and the client's bullshit radar starts to go off. Less than three and it does not have enough impact to last beyond the meeting. **Many clients are very nervous when they first meet an escort**. Remember, this is something you do on a regular basis but for most clients visiting an escort is a treat which they can only enjoy every now and again. As an escort you have to take control and make the client comfortable. One very quick way to do this is to take off your shoes as soon as you can, although this may sound irrelevant this one simple act will send a very positive signal to the client that you are willing to take the lead, this will take pressure off of him and the nerves will just flood away.

If he is visiting you, offer him a drink. Sit down with him; make interesting and vaguely suggestive conversation, in other words, flirt with him, turn him on; kiss him. This should take about 10–15 minutes. Then suggest that perhaps he, or both of you together, take a shower. This can be fun, ensures that he is clean and not smelling bad, gets you naked easily and at this point has taken you as near as dammit to halfway

The Reality of Escorting

through your hour. Soap him down playfully, tease his cock and balls, lightly scratch his back – get him going. From Georgina who says she orgasms with nearly every client:

> I never spend time with a client without making him shower first. I don't care if he says he showered 15 minutes earlier. I also buy a new toothbrush for every client that visits me. I cannot bear men that are minging. It is the ultimate turn-off!

Then towel him down and back to the bedroom, or wherever it is that the 'action' is going to take place. Ideally you will have discussed your client's sexual requirements with him on the phone and will already have worked out your own 'time scenario' based on those requirements. A few clients only want to pleasure you. They will want to lick you out and masturbate you till you orgasm. Most clients however see your paid role as one of pleasuring them. Quite often this will start with cock sucking.

Do not have unprotected oral sex if you have cuts or ulcers in or on your mouth or any kind of gum infection. Don't do it without being aware of all the risks. Just because other people do it does not mean that you have to, make the choice for yourself. Never be coerced into doing anything you do not want to do.

If you don't do O/WO (oral sex without a condom) place a condom on his cock – doing so with your mouth, if you have learnt how, never fails to impress – and give him the best blowjob he has ever had. Escorts tend to fall into two camps on this issue. Half of them would rather suck cock because if they can make a guy orgasm that way then they may not have to perform penetrative sex. The other half are the same part of the female population who just cannot get their sexual heads around having a cock in their mouth. It's a personal preference thing.

Oral sex is a big issue. O/WO became a much bigger issue for clients as a result of the social changes that arose from AIDS and the definitive need for safe sex, particularly among sex workers. There is a feeling by the client that they are getting something extra with O/WO, particularly in England and America where many clients will reject a girl who does not perform O/WO.

It would seem that in Australia the accepted practice is to use a condom for everything – oral, anal and vaginal – and in the 2003 edition of the STD Handbook published by the Australian Government Info Access Network they even recommend using latex gloves for hand jobs. It has also become the accepted practice in Australian brothels for sex workers to check their clients for STDs before servicing them. In New South Wales, Australia, the local government health department says:

> The decision about whether or not to engage in oral sex is a personal one dependant on a person accept-ing this minimal risk of transmitting HIV. Use of a condom or dental dam reduces this small risk further. However it should be noted that unprotected oral sex may be an efficient way to transmit other STDs.[1]

The Reality of Escorting

It is always ultimately your choice. There is a degree of risk. International AIDS charity AVERT gives the following information:

The risk of HIV transmission from an infected partner through oral sex is much smaller than the risk of HIV transmission from anal or vaginal sex. Because of this, measuring the exact risk of HIV transmission as a result of oral sex is very difficult. In addition, since most sexually active individuals practise oral sex in addition to other forms of sex, such as vaginal and/or anal sex, when transmission occurs, it is difficult to determine whether or not it occurred as a result of oral sex or other more risky sexual activities. Finally, several co-factors can increase the risk of HIV transmission through oral sex, including: oral ulcers, bleeding gums, genital sores and the presence of other STDs.

When scientists describe the risk of transmitting an infectious disease, like HIV, the term 'theoretical risk' is often used. Very simply, 'theoretical risk' means that passing an infection from one person to another is possible, even though there may not yet be any actual documented cases. 'Theoretical risk' is not the same as likelihood. In other words, stating that HIV infection is 'theoretically possible' does not necessarily mean it is likely to happen – only that it might. Documented risk, on the other hand, is used to describe transmission that has actually occurred, been investigated, and documented in the scientific literature.

In Good Company

Various scientific studies have been performed around the world to try and document and study instances of HIV transmission through oral sex. A programme in San Francisco studied 198 people, nearly all gay or bisexual men. The subjects stated that they had only had oral sex for a year, from six months preceding the six-month study to its end. 20 per cent of the study participants, 39 people, reported performing oral sex on partners they knew to be HIV positive. 35 of those did not use a condom and 16 reported swallowing cum. No-one became HIV positive during the study. Due to the low number of unprotected serodiscordant pairings, all that can be said is that there was a less than 2.8 per cent chance of infection through oral sex over a year.[2]

This shows us that the risk is most definitely there so, forgive me for being repetitive, don't do it if you don't like it. Don't do it if you have cuts or ulcers on or in your mouth or any kind of gum infection. Don't do it without being aware of all the risks. Just because other people do it does not mean that you have to; make the choice for yourself. Never be coerced into doing anything you do not want to do. The same applies to CIM (cum in mouth). If you like swallowing semen, great. If you don't enjoy it and have not analysed the risks for yourself, don't do it. Many clients will reject a girl because she won't indulge in letting him come into her mouth. My advice to girls who will do O/WO but don't allow CIM is to tell the client that you might, if you like

The Reality of Escorting

him. After all, swallowing a man's spunk is a very personal thing. Then, if you are doing your job well enough, you can get him to shoot his load somewhere else. Personally I think that clients who insist on this are being very unrealistic. While many women will do almost everything else, CIM seems to be one of those things that crosses a mental barrier most women do not seem to want to leap, as Ruslana, an escort for several years, shows us:

> I do anal, I do almost anything, but I can't and won't do O/WO and definitely not CIM . . . it's just icky!

Another thing to be aware of with oral sex is not to let yourself be coerced into overdoing it, as Nicki was:

> The client booked me initially for two hours. When I got there he told me he only wanted oral sex – no penetration. Great, I thought. After the two hours he produced another £300 and asked if I would stay for longer, I phoned the agency and I agreed to stay. Anyway, I sucked his cock constantly for six hours and left. The next day I woke up and my tongue muscle was torn and I had severe whiplash – I was unable to work for a week!

So you have sucked his cock, or not, and it is time to get down to the brass tacks – penetration. Put a condom on him. Always make sure it is fresh from a new, unopened, date-checked pack. (Condoms have use-by dates as well!) Vaginal penetrative sex is the norm. Whatever position you choose is between him and you.

If you do 'A' or A-Levels (anal) or Greek, as the Americans call it, then make sure you use a fresh condom for anal penetration. Anal sex, like oral sex without a condom, is totally a personal preference. Do not do it with a client if you have never done it before with a previous partner. Do not do it with a client if you do not like it. Do not do it with a client if he has a huge penis. Female rectums can get very used to penetrative sex but it has to be done gently and lovingly, which is not something you should expect from a man who is paying you for sex. Some men want anal because what they really want is sex with another man. Some men want anal penetration over and above vaginal penetration because they somehow feel it eases their guilt about having sex with an escort at all. Some men want anal sex because they come from cultures where, as teenagers, anal sex with other boys is preferable to taking the virginity of a girl one is not married to. Some men want anal sex because they want to hurt the woman. Some men want anal because they have been exposed to a constant diet of porn and think that this is what they are supposed to be doing. Some men, and women, just like it.

As discussed in Chapter Two, a small amount of clients have a fetish or perversion that can only be fulfilled, for a variety of reasons already touched on, by paying someone to indulge those fantasies. BDSM is the most common term for this (bondage, domination and sadomasochism). Being either dominant or submissive to order is something to be approached seriously. Just like O/WO and A – only get involved in these things if you want to. Do not let anyone tie you up if it is going to make you feel uncomfortable. Being a submissive can be delicious but it can also be fraught with dangers – both physical and psychological – and I believe it is not wise to experiment with your sexuality on this level with clients. Do not tie anyone up unless you know what you are doing. Do not indulge in extremes of role play (above and beyond the role play that enables you to escort successfully) if they make you uncomfortable. If you do indulge in these 'games' make sure that you both have an agreed 'safe' word so that if either party wants things to stop it does so immediately. Unless you are supremely confident, and experienced, I would suggest not indulging in these activities with a client you have only just met for the first time. If a first-time client asks you when you actually meet him if you would play a little S&M game with him, tell him – if you are inclined to go there – that you might if your first encounter with him goes well so to wait for your next meeting. This serves two purposes. One is that you are leading him into re-booking you. The second is that it gives him something to think on – it tantalises. Men quite often, like children, want more of that which they are temporarily forbidden.

Self-Protection

As an escort you are in effect self-employed. While any reputable agency will run security checks, metaphorically watch your back and get work for you, your own security reality is primarily down to you. There are many ways in which you can guard against a lot of the pitfalls sex workers encounter.

Always practise safe sex, that is, always use condoms. There is never an excuse not to. If a client says he cannot perform with a condom, have absolutely nothing to do with him and inform your agency immediately. Have regular check-ups at a reputable STI (Sexually Transmitted Infections) clinic. Condoms, while being the best form of protection we have against disease, are not 100 per cent reliable and accidents like condoms splitting do happen so get yourself checked out every three months. Believe me, doing this simple thing on a regular basis will give you piece of mind. In England and Australia, these clinics are free of charge and are quite often in the forefront of research into sexually transmitted diseases and so encourage sex workers to use their services without fear of exposure or condemnation. (Also, in England all STI clinics provide free condoms, in Australia most sell condoms at a reduced rate to sex workers and in America it varies from state to state – some do, some don't.) Be assured that at all these clinics your confidentiality is always respected.

While for the most part clients are decent people who would not dream of hurting anyone, there are, like any sub-group of the population, one or two exceptions to the rule. Hopefully you will never encounter this either in your work or day-to-day life, but let us be realistic – it happens. It is better to be prepared than to be sorry afterwards. Gemma's story highlights a particular horror that could have been dealt with differently.

I don't really know where to start. It's quite embarrassing for me to tell this story because looking back on it, it should never have happened. I had a dog – a big black dog and my flatmate, Honey, in the flat. It was my flat. Maybe that's why I am writing this – so girls reading this book will know what not to do. It probably would have been different if my flatmate and me had not been arguing and I was feeling vulnerable and incapable anyway. You shouldn't work when you are in that kind of a state – but that is easier said than done when you are in need of the money.

Anyway my agent called me with an incall. These days I would never work from my own home, but at that time I was 17 and me and Honey wanted to make as much money as possible. The guy came round. He actually asked on the phone if I lived with anyone and I pretended I didn't. Honey and I always pretended there was no one else there, I don't know why, but I think for most clients it's a privacy thing. We also hid the dog, in case he didn't like dogs – I had lost a client once because he was scared of our dog, but thinking about it now it's so stupid to put the client before your own safety. Anyway I took the guy into the room and at first it was all fine. He wasn't very into talking – but to be honest when they came to my house I wanted them out as soon as possible. We kissed and everything seemed fine until it came to putting the condom on. He wouldn't let me. He kept pushing my hands away and saying 'no, no'. I said that we had to and I tried again and then he got my wrists and pulled them off him. He put them up beside my head. I was still holding the condom in one hand. I didn't even struggle, I don't know why. I was really scared. I didn't shout either. I knew that Honey was out there but I didn't have enough in me to shout. It wasn't fear that was stopping me. It was shame. I was so violated and ashamed and powerless. All my control had been grabbed from me. As he was fucking me I was just whispering in his ear: 'please stop, please stop – can we just put the condom on.' I was thinking, God, please don't let him have AIDS. But I was strangely calm, I didn't move, I kind of accepted that this was my fate. I didn't feel anything after a while. Everything shut off. I remember his hands on my wrists; I remember his shoulder and his weight. He had dark greying hair and sunspots. I can still feel the rhythm of him. But I can't remember his face. It is blank, it's blurred, I can't remember it at all. I remember the feeling of him cumming – that was the first time anyone had come inside me. I didn't like it. He kissed me on the forehead. Then I don't remember him leaving, I don't know what happened. I don't think he threatened me, I think he just left. I remember him going though. Everything kind of flooded back into me, it was like I held my breath and then started breathing again. I felt like I should be upset so I tried to cry. You expect to feel one way and you just don't. I couldn't cry, I felt dulled.

I told Honey and she said that it was karma and I deserved it – because I had slept with someone she had once had a threesome with a few days before. That was it, I didn't tell anyone else. I didn't tell my agent – which was really bad because that man should have been blacklisted. I didn't tell the police because I was underage. I also didn't see it as rape. He had come there and paid for it, to me it wasn't as if I was grabbed in a back ally. I didn't know so I just moved on from it. I got checked and I was okay. Honey made me go and get the coil so I couldn't get pregnant. That was it.

A few months later I had what I think was a flashback. The biggest effect it had on me is that for a long time after that I wasn't able to come. I lost all my trust in sex. Even now with my girlfriend I find it hard not to be in control. I don't know, it was something that I blocked off for such a long time, I am not sure if I ever really dealt with it. It feels like a film to me. The colours of my bedroom are more vivid than any other memory I have of that room. But there are whole chunks I can't remember. I just dis-connected from it, after all I had to keep working, I had to sleep in that room, I had to get on with my life like nothing had happened. I would say to anyone wanting to work, that if you do it – do it properly. You do this job for yourself so make sure you put yourself and your safety first. Check the guys out; let them know you have a job, etc. You don't owe these men anything and you don't have to do anything. After that night it took me a long time to learn to say 'no' assertively. It's your body and you should always respect it. I was lucky, I didn't catch any diseases but that was complete luck. Gambling as an escort is foolish and dangerous.

It is illegal to escort if you are under 18 years of age.

There are some old-fashioned but very obvious things you can do to protect yourself. Always carry a spray bottle or can of strong, preferably cheap and nasty smelling per-fume, hairspray or other substance that you can then shoot or spray into your attacker's eyes. This will not hurt your attacker in any big way but it will give you that extra moment's head start to get away from him. Also being doused in something noxious will mean that he has to get cleaned up or have people notice that something is not quite right with him. In England, Mace is illegal but in

The Reality of Escorting

America, France, Spain, Italy and Holland it is easily available and many women use it for self-defence.

Learn how to kick a man where it really hurts – his balls. Practise with a girlfriend and a pillow till you can kick as hard as you possibly can without hesitation – it is the hesitation that sometimes makes this solution a drawback. Another good tactic which will leave him much less able to persist in assaulting you is, if you are wearing stiletto heels, while not great for running away, you can bring your stiletto heel down hard onto his foot between the first and second metatarsals and grind. Very very hard. (This also works on men on public transport who use the sardine-like conditions to inappropriately fondle and touch women without express prior permission.)

The main thing is not to show any fear. Do not hesitate. Use your brain. Never allow yourself to be locked in a room where you cannot get out of your own volition. Always know your exits and always have a 'change of plan' strategy. Always have the wherewithal to get yourself home (remember Becky's story from Chapter Two, page 57). Finally, stay fit. Work out at home or the gym, learn a martial art (I know more sex workers who do kickboxing than any other profession) or take a self-defence course. Take as much control as you can over what happens to your body on every level. One more thing to keep in mind is sleep. Get lots of sleep. If you overdo it and are too exhausted your reaction times are down, your brain is slower, your natural instincts become foggy and you open your immune system up for destruction. For the same reasons keep your alcohol and drug intake to a minimum, particularly when you are on call or with a client.

The other potential danger with clients is giving away too much of yourself. We have seen in previous case studies how dangerous and disturbing this can be. It is in your own self-interest and protection to keep the real you and your escort alter ego as separate as possible. Some clients, very few admittedly, do become obsessed with the girls they see. If you suspect that this is happening to you, tell your agency about it immediately. An ethical agent will gently try to dissuade the client from seeing you again and will recommend another girl to him. Or they will lie and just say you are not available. They cannot do this though if they do not know about it. So be honest and upfront for your own safety and protection.

If you work from a flat neither you nor your agency should give the client your address until he is five to ten minutes away from you and his booked appointment time. This means that he cannot just turn up when you are not prepared for him. This will not stop a client from becoming over-interested after he has seen you but will alleviate some of the creepy types who just like collecting sex workers' addresses. (Yes, these guys exist!)

If you have created an alter ego stick with her. If she is a student but you are really a single mother do not start talking about your kids. If you are Polish but say that you are Russian make sure that you can speak the language. If you are worried about your friends and family seeing you on the internet, make sure your face is blurred or removed altogether. Keep your real life wrapped up safe and away from clients.

The Reality of Escorting

Finally there is the issue of entrapment. The legal definition of entrapment is 'where a police officer or other law enforcement officer induces a person to commit a crime that the person wouldn't have committed otherwise for the purpose of bringing a criminal prosecution against that person.'[3]

It doesn't happen often but it does happen. Mandy, who worked in a massage parlour in Auckland, New Zealand before decriminalisation, tells us what happened to her:

> A guy walked into the massage parlour where I worked. Obviously at the time I did not know that he was a policeman. He paid his $20 for a massage, which I gave him. When I had finished the massage he asked me for 'extras', this is the common term used for sex, not unusual in my line of work. I winked at him and asked him for $60. I even called him 'Sir'. Within seconds the parlour was crawling with police, they burst in and arrested everyone in the place – clients and girls. I was charged with being a common prostitute and was taken to court. I told the court that the policeman had asked for sex, that I had not offered it – which indeed I hadn't – no explicit sexual terms or phrases were used and that this was a case of entrapment. The judge agreed with me and let me go.

In Good Company

This not only applies to the sex worker but also to the client, as Henry's story shows:

> I was cruising round Central London looking for nothing in particular. A girl, dressed for sex, was standing on a well-known-for-prostitute-girls street corner. I approached her with a view to sex. I was gobsmacked and dismayed to find out that this cute little thing was in fact a policewoman working undercover! I went to court and got a fine despite arguing that it had been entrapment. If that particular girl had not been where she was, looking like she did I would not have committed this so-called offence.

While sex work is *not* illegal in the UK, soliciting is. Kerb-crawling is seen as the client soliciting and was Henry's undoing.

How we as escorts avoid this is simple. If you ever have a booking with more than one client at the same time, whether it is a male and female couple or two men, you only ever take the money off one of them, in a room with just the two of you. There cannot be a third party involved in the exchange of cash because what you are selling is not your body but your time. That way, should anything occur, like police entrapment, it is your word against the one person who gave you the money. If a third party had been present and you had actually stated that the money you were receiving was for sex, then that third party could testify against you in court. If a client will not agree to this there is a small chance that he or she is in fact a representative of the law. There is more about escorting and the law in Chapter Six.

Cash

The overwhelming reason why we do this is the cash. As previously stated, you always get your fee at the start of the booking. No exceptions, as Becky's story on page 57 shows us. We take cash and only cash because cheques bounce and credit cards take commission. Besides, carrying a credit card machine around with you is tiresome for all but the most successful. Generally only take cash in the currency of where you live, though any good agency will be able to do a currency convert for you in seconds. Vicki's story explains why:

> I was a student in London; I was very naïve and very broke. I did a little escorting. I got a job with a Bangladeshi man in a rich house in Hampstead. He paid me 1,074 Bangladeshi taka. It seemed like a lot of money. I did the job. When I phoned the agency and told them, they did a currency convert. My taka equalled £9. I was gutted!

Anything other than cash is a freebie. Value yourself higher. Do not work for an agency that claims its clients pay them by cheque therefore they will pay you by cheque when the client's cheque clears. You will get ripped off.

In Good Company

Tipping by clients is of course totally acceptable and is to be encouraged. If, on top of your fee, he gives you flowers or perfume or your cab fare home take it graciously but do not make the mistake of thinking that this pays for extra 'no cash' time with you. On the other hand, charging over and above the agreed fee for 'extra services' (like anal or BDSM) unless agreed on the phone before meeting is not on. Many girls get a bad reputation for, in effect, squeezing money for favours out of clients. This hurts the whole industry. Charge an agreed fee, give good service and keep it simple.

Be wary, once you have been paid, of leaving your cash and belongings alone with the client. Most clients as I have said are decent people but one or two are not, as Lucia points out:

> I met a client in his hotel, he paid me, we did the business, I went to the loo just before leaving, I came out, picked up my bag and left. When I got down to the street and checked my bag I only had a few notes in there – he had taken the bulk of my money.

The moral of that story: always take your cash with you. Also make sure you check your fee when he first gives it. Do it discreetly and politely but check it. Joanna's story highlights why:

> I had spoken to the client a few times on the phone and he seemed really nice. He came to see me at

my flat and appeared incredibly nervous. I soon found out why. He gave me an envelope with the cash. I took it to the bedroom, closed the door and opened the envelope. There was one genuine £20 note on top, the rest were all bad fakes. I was so angry. Did this guy think I was stupid? Did he really think I would let him fuck me for £20?!!? I opened the door and he was standing right there. I asked him to leave and he got verbally aggressive with me, like I was the one who had done something wrong. In the end I called the police and he left.

This doesn't happen very often but it does happen. Be aware. We live in a cold calculating world where, sometimes, bad things do occur. Minimise the chances of that happening to you by being on the ball, aware, thorough and careful.

What you do with your cash afterwards is down to you but I strongly advise that you save at least half of it. Remember that part of what you are selling is your youth and beauty. Inevitably, these fade. The work will lessen. As Kylie says:

Escorting is hard work, physically, spiritually and mentally. You had better be sure you have something to show for your time and your money because at the end of the day this is not going to last forever.

In Good Company

If you spend your twenties blowing all your money on clothes, shoes, drugs (none of which I would recommend) or whatever your personal passion is, then when the escorting runs out what have you got to show for it? You can either stash your cash under the bed or you can put it into a bank. If you choose to put it into a bank I suggest you get yourself a good accountant and register yourself with your taxation office as a freelance entertainer, model or masseuse. Pay your taxes every year, just like everyone else and invest your earnings in assets – like property, or stocks and shares, or your children's education. How you deal with it is entirely up to you.

The last part of the cash 'circle' is paying your commission to an agency. Many agencies like you to bring them your commission immediately after completion of the job and some will not give you another job until you have done so. The motivation for this is mistrust and greed. Some will give you their bank account details and ask you to bank at your nearest branch of their bank the following day. Both of these are usual and, whatever the previously agreed arrangement is, should always be honoured unless the agency has let you down in some way. Not giving the agency its commission as soon as you can may also mean that you miss your next job. The only thing that is not acceptable is the agency taking your fee, removing their commission and then paying you after the job has been completed.

The Reality of Escorting

Friends and Family

If you have decided to embark on this life with your alter
ego totally hidden from your friends and family it can be a
lonely though, more often than not, safe path. Many people are ambivalent about sex work until they know it is their
daughter or sister or girlfriend who is doing it – think back
to Andrew's comment in Chapter Two (page 39). Letting
people in your 'real' life know what you do can be fraught
with anguish and disaster. The best friend you had for years
who seemed so open-minded but who now won't speak to
you because you confessed your secret double life to her is
a common thread for many sex workers. It is, in my opinion, far better to keep your lives totally separate, though it
is not easy. Keep your working profile as far removed from
your real existence as you can possibly manage. Find a good
excuse to be looking good and leaving soon. 'Promotions' or
PR work is a good fall back for this. It covers a variety of
actions and looks and is really only half a lie. Where this
falls down is for the single mother. Single mums have to
have a reliable back up for their kids. The very nature of
escorting means that some jobs come in without the
required notice to book a babysitter. The best way round
this is to find another escort who is a single mum and share
the load. As Kate did:

> I'm a single mother of two. Both my parents are
> dead and both fathers of my children abandoned
> them not long after their respective births. I am a

good and loving mother. I became friendly with another escort single mother and we child-mind for each other when we go out on jobs. This means that both sets of children are always cared for, that there is enough money for everything that me and my children need in order to live in a decent way and I get to spend as much time as I need with my kids. Because of the kids I couldn't keep a proper job going. I had no support network as such. This was the only choice I felt I could make.

Remember lovers and day-job employers are not likely to understand why you need to escort in order to buy that new car that your job won't quite cover and your man hasn't the spare cash to buy for you.

If you choose to share your working life with those people around you who are important to you, make sure that they are strong enough emotionally in themselves to cope with what you do, as Chrissie, the girlfriend of an escort, explains:

I understand why Lauren has to do it but I don't like it, it makes me feel sick to my bones. When I am home waiting for her to come back from a job all sorts runs through my head: I start thinking – is she enjoying it? Are they making her come? Then I feel like an arsehole cos I am thinking hell! No! How can any lesbian enjoy that? Then I start freaking out about her safety – I panic and call her phone worrying that she is being gang-raped or murdered or abused. I can't sleep till she is home. It's made worse if it's late, between three and six in the morning, because at that time I can't just jump on a train and come get her. If she is busy she can't answer the phone and that freaks me out. I ring and ring till she answers which puts her in a mood – cos she's doing her job – but what am I meant to do? I can't stand her being near me when she comes back cos she smells of them if she hasn't had a shower yet. I just don't like it – it fucks me up and gives me nightmares. I can't even handle writing any more because I have to shut it in the back of my mind so I don't have to think of it – if I did it would drive me mad. And her and me would argue. In the past both of us have taken loads of drugs to cope. But now we are much better we don't put ourselves through it very often. This summer Lauren is going to get out of debt and then it will be over forever.

Many couples survive one person working in the sex industry but many more do not.

Never enter the industry to assuage the sexual or financial desires of your partner. If you do share this part of your life with someone else then be aware of the associative impact that what you do for a living has on his or her life and be prepared for the fallout. Many men, while being happy to benefit from the profits of sex work, are not so keen on the actual reality of how that money is acquired.

In Good Company

See Marilyn's story in Chapter Five (page 119) for a stripper's take on sex industry earnings and partners.

It is a double life and being single-minded and a good actress helps to maintain that duality, but if you are caught out (as mentioned in Chapter One) – bluff it out. Lie. People have a tendency to believe what they want to. If your 'real' life is so obviously not that of the sex worker why shouldn't people believe your denial? Natalie, who worked for an international bank, tells what happened to her:

I had been with the company for about two years and had been turned down for promotion, and the extra salary that goes with it, twice in six months. I decided to do some escorting. I registered with two agencies and my pictures went up on their websites. I managed the two things successfully for another six months until my mother died and I took one month's compassionate leave from my job. In the third week of being off work my supervisor emailed me to say that they had seen my pictures on the internet and that I was being called in for a disciplinary hearing. At first I freaked out completely. I phoned the agencies and asked them to remove my images immediately, which they both did, and one advised me to pretend outrage at the suggestion that I would do such a thing. I telephoned my supervisor and told her how upset and appalled I was that she could even think that I was that sort of woman. The whole experience was incredibly disturbing, particularly as I was grieving at the time, and I decided to hand in my resignation, which the company accepted. I changed my escort name and photos and I now escort full-time.

Things You Don't Have To Do

Although I have said it before, I do not think it can be reiterated enough. Never do anything that makes you feel uncomfortable. With agencies this means everything from the casting couch blowjob to being coerced, or even forced, into seeing a client you are uncomfortable with. From doing a freebie for your agent's mates to 'performing' with other girls when you are not genuinely bisexual. Sophie's story shows this:

> My English was not very good and the agent he ask me if I like girls and I say yes of course I like girls but I did not understand what he mean. That night he sends me to hotel with other girl and she tries to touch me. I try to explain to her and she is very nice but agent not give me jobs anymore.

All of these things are patently wrong. Have enough strength and self-respect to say no and mean it. The same thing applies to an agency that you feel takes too large a percentage of your fee. Just say no and walk away. Do not let anyone control your existence any more than the state and life already does.

Chapter Four

A Day in the Life of . . .

Now is the time to hear it from the whore's mouth, so to speak. These are four very different women's lives in their own words. Debbie is a full-time student who escorts evenings and weekends and supports herself and her education through escorting. Her story is somewhat harrowing for one so young. Joy is a restaurant manager who escorts whenever her shifts permit and is saving to buy her own restaurant. Marysia is a full-time independent escort who has bought a house from the proceeds of sex work. She is intelligent, successful and fully in control of her own existence. Lyn works a gruelling schedule in the brothels of Queensland. These are their own stories in their own words.

Debbie's Story

I wake up, get ready for college and walk the dog. Then I commute across London to where my college is. I love my course, I could not get through juggling everything like this with out loving it. I spend the whole day at college – our hours are quite varied though: 9–5, 12–6, 9–1. It is strange being at college. Everyone around me seems so young, they still live with their parents and their lives seem so simple compared to mine. I feel so jealous that they can properly commit to the course. I want to be like them, I want to be healthy and fresh and fit in. It is hard to be like them because my life is so far away from them. I can't go out to the pub on Friday because I have to work. I am supporting someone else and working full-time as an escort, I hardly ever take time off. On the train to school I text the agents telling them my hours for the night. Then I switch into college mode – it is not always easy because I have to call agents in school from the toilet when they want me to arrange a job for later. Once I was really scared because my phone rang in class and the teacher had a habit of answering the person's phone as punishment for disturbing his class. I thought the school was going to find out and I'd get kicked out. But fortunately it wasn't an agent calling.

After college it takes me about an hour and a half to get home. Then I go back into escort mode. I buy the food shopping, walk the dog, clean the flat, eat and bathe and get ready to work. My agents always insist that I am ready to leave if I get a call so I get dressed in my work clothes and get made up. I do my coursework like that which is always very strange – you don't relax easily when you are waiting for work. I also often get offered a job before I am ready – but you don't turn work down so there is a mad rush between the call and the cab coming. My flatmate and I wait for work doing coursework, eating or watching a film. The calls always seem to come just as I am sitting down to eat, so often I have to leave my food. Unfortunately if you are full-time at college and escorting you have to be signed on and available for work while you do other things – because there are not enough hours in the day. I usually get a job between 8 and midnight. The midnight ones are awful because you get to the job for one, spend an hour there and get home by three, if it's an hour, but sometimes I don't get home till five/six. That means washing, dog-walking and falling straight to bed to catch a few hours of sleep to then get up for college. If I don't get a job by one, then I go to sleep, wake up at four and sign on with the late night agencies. When I do those jobs I come straight home, change for college and go. It's exhausting. I am so often late from simply oversleeping that I had to tell my college what was going on – they were actually really supportive – but I think they feel it is a waste because I could do so much better at college if I had enough sleep. Three hours or less sleep a night takes its toll – I don't really know how I do it apart from the fact that I have to.

It is actually really hard to describe a typical outcall – every time is different. But, for example, my agent called me and got me to call a man called Steven back. I did, he was quite chatty and seemed friendly. He wanted to know all the usual information about what I looked like and what I was prepared to do – or in his words 'what can we do in this hour?' 'How do I know you're fit?' – he was quite easy to talk with. He had obviously hired girls before. He gave me his address in Highbury and told me to come over. I called the agent back and had a bit of a mad rush to get ready before the cab came because I had only just signed on – you have to look beautiful, dressed-up, made-up and sexy. I get cabs to houses because you need to be there quick and they can be quite hard to find. Once I arrived Steve and I said our hellos – he was English and about 45, I think, and he said I was beautiful and kissed me on the cheek. I then explained to him that I have to let my agent know I am here so could I please take the money. He got the money and offered me a glass of wine. After I counted the money and called my agent to say everything was fine, we sat on his sofa and talked and drank wine. Just kind of friendly talk about what he did for a living – he was a designer. He was nice but I could tell he didn't have lots of money and would only want an hour. You have to be on the ball to be a good escort – you have to please lots of different types of people and to do that you have to know what they want. After about 20 minutes he kissed me then invited me to his bedroom. We undressed and kissed each other and he was very keen to make me come. After he did (or thought he did) I gave him a bj, which he really liked, and we had sex in several different positions before he came. Just to let you know, girls have to bring their own protection. After we were done – it was quite quick – we talked and hugged until it was time for me to call my agent. I offered him another hour but he didn't have any more money. So he ordered me a cab and I took a quick shower. We said our goodbyes and agreed he would call me again. I suppose this is your standard one-hour job with a certain quite common type of client. I call these jobs 'polite, middle-class, easy jobs'. They are nice but sometimes you don't clear that much money after the cabs and agency fees – if it's far you can usually get the guy to pay for the cab. These kinds of jobs are nearly always in the evening – I think the kind of jobs you get can depend on what time you sign on.

Life is non-stop but I am juggling about seven agents, most of whom want you to be on all the time and expect fees to be paid into the bank. Then there's college, caring for my girlfriend Amanda and everything else. I sometimes get stress rashes and sometimes I don't eat because I am so busy that I actually forget to. But the worst is the double life aspect – it is maddening at times and upsetting and isolating – you have to be strong in your self to be able to cope with that part of it, you have to lie to people you love and be prepared not to be understood.

But it is worth it, I have learnt a lot during this time of my life and I am determined not to leave college. I am so grateful I haven't given up college to become a full-time escort because it makes me feel secure about the future, which escorting can't give you.

A Day in the Life of . . .

Joy's Story

It's 6 am and, even though I didn't get home last night until 3 am, I am up. Yoga time; peace, no one is up and London is still quiet. I have a very heavy day ahead; I try to melt three lives into one. My work at the restaurant, my social life, my escort life. I have three wardrobes, three sets of 'friends', three personalities. I guess it's a perfect life if you are a schizophrenic.

Although my heart is in the restaurant, I need the escorting to make the restaurant dream happen.

9 am, I open the restaurant and prepare for a busy sunny day.

The weirdest thing about escorting is that sometimes when I am at the restaurant, I look at some customers and think, 'he could be a client', and I am sure that if he uses the escorting services, he would think, 'I wonder if she would'. Anybody could.

I don't have to pretend when I am at the restaurant, but what is really hard for me is to pretend to be naïve or without a strong opinion while I am 'entertaining' a client, because my personality is dormant then. I can't tell them, 'Shut the fuck up, you are boring me with your lies and promises!!!' Because they always do.

The worst thing is not being able to tell my friends, mainly because I would have to give them an explanation, but the words will not capture exactly why it is that I chose escorting as a means to an end. It always comes out as an overused cliché, we are not all victims. But I promised myself, if one of them asks me then I won't lie. So far no one has dared.

Lunchtime is over and my mobile is on because I know I have a dinner date tonight, a regular . . . I have a couple of them and it's the best of the worst as they get to know you a little so the pretence is not so much, and they say they want to help. But I only want the money so I can raise enough to open my own place some day. Some of them offered to lend me a large amount but I know there will be something heftier to pay, besides I don't want them in my life long-term! They'll think I owe them!

So 10.30 pm I rush out of the restaurant, I have a change of clothes, take a cab and off to a hotel in Regents Park, not too far. I would prefer staying late at the restaurant and having a drink with my staff but . . . maybe tomorrow.

When I decide I am going to spend the evening out, then I will not escort.

I use to socialise with other working girls but we would be out and the phone would ring, and they couldn't say no. I feel sorry for them, for me they are slaves.

So, in the hotel, shower, then pre-dinner sex, I need to remember what lies I told him last time. Then dinner, I don't like to be open with them, there is no price for that, and I want all of them to know that. In the meantime, every time I go to a restaurant or bar I need to make sure I don't know anybody there, cos after working for over ten years in London restaurants, you get to know pretty much every one, again I've never got caught.

The other thing is, I can't really show off my food and

wine knowledge, cos that may make him feel insecure; he booked an escort so he could feel good, have light conversation, smiles, me being impressed by him, and blah blah blah. Sex, that's the most important. And when we get back to the room, after an hour or so, he's asleep and I can sneak out!

Yeah!!! Free!!! Good night!!!

I've got time to change, again, and meet some friends for a drink or two.

So that will be it for this week, I don't want to do this more than twice a week.

I wonder if the cab driver knows?

Marysia's Story

Most days, unless my phone is switched off for a very good reason or I'm out of town, I am 'on-call'. Usually up until about 10 pm. I really don't like to do bookings much later than that, but I will if I have plenty of notice or the client sounds especially nice.

Not working late is partly a safety issue and partly it's the people you get later in the evening . . . In my experience most people who call after 10.30 are usually half pissed or probably cokeheads and I won't deal with either thank you! Many a time I've turned my work phone on in the morning, only to receive some random text or message from a guy sounding oddly 'perky' for 4.30 am. 'Hi, my name's Alan – I'm in Wandsworth' and can I give him a call if I'm still up. Definite cokehead. You can hear it in their voices. Not a chance. I'm always well tucked up at that time of night in any case, and even if I were still up, I wouldn't go. They are usually incredibly annoying city boys with overinflated egos, sticking what remains of their last bonus up their nose. It's never a smooth transaction. Either they are rude or don't want to pay or they want you to stay half the night when they only booked for an hour or they can't get it up and you have to wank them for hours or *something*. It's just way more hassle than it's worth.

I do have one regular who *always* wants to see me after 10.30 pm and it's *always* 'last minute', but with him it's okay. I like him a lot. He works horrendous hours and it's the only time he can see me. I've noted he always has a rucksack with him and wears very good quality walking shoes and looks like he's just about to embark on an expedition of some sort. He also likes to take the piss out of himself, which is hilarious and he always brings a really nice bottle of wine, which he practically downs in one. This suits me fine as I hardly drink.

I like to get up at 8 am. Morning time is my time. Before work time. Usually. You may get the very odd occasion when a client is especially keen to see you, but for whatever reason can't do a more normal time and can only make it at 8 or 9 am. Before they go into the office. 'I'm in a meeting', they say. That's fine.

A quick shower and then my phone goes on. I immediately delete any random/unintelligible/rude texts from my work phone and call anyone leaving a genuine-sounding message. Next I write my list for the day.

A Day in the Life of . . .

This list has everything important that I need/want to do in the near future. At the moment it reads:

1. **Organise all for photo shoot**. Very important, and takes a shitload of thought and planning. Good pictures are the main selling point in this industry it seems, and although I have lots of great ones it's always good to have new stuff up there. I could use fakes but I prefer the real deal.

2. **£330 to Eros**. Eros is a huge site I currently advertise on. I'm trying to maximise my exposure by doing some extra advertising with them. Will be interesting to see if the extra money pays off.

3. **New additions to my website**. For this I need a whole day and my friend Dez. I have lots of new pics of friends and a couple of guys I want to put on, plus quite a few text changes and maybe a new couple of pages. It might be useful to have a FAQ's section and a 'first-timers guide'. My personal favourite new addition is going to be 'client etiquette' which will most definitely include the *no onions* clause. Some people!

4. **Write script for video clip**. I haven't seen it on many sites yet and thought a short video clip might be fun on my site. It gives clients a chance to see my 'stunning central London apartment' and hear my voice. Which is nice I've been told. I'm not too keen on having my face all over the web so we'll have to be clever with the filming. Perhaps I'll stay out of the clip altogether and just do a voice over . . .

In Good Company

By this point I've probably had a couple of withheld numbers calling. These I don't entertain for more than about 30 seconds and I'm very firm about that. People who withhold their numbers are nine times out of ten messing around/ jerking off or want to abuse you. If they are genuine they will call back showing their number. End of story. Then I hit the gym. A chore more than anything else but you do feel fabulous afterwards. Then it's time to eat, take my vitamins, chuck on some make-up and I'm ready to start the day!

Bookings mainly happen in the evening but you do get the 'lunchtime crowd' who come rushing across town in a black cab, clutching a briefcase to have a spot of midday fun. These I like. The block of flats where I work is always dead in the daytime – everyone who lives there is out working so I feel like I have the whole place to myself. I absolutely love the building. It has a huge shiny green front door and a very large, airy entrance hall with a beautiful old mirror on the right, leading you up an enormous sweeping flight of stairs. The banisters are dark and sturdy and there are massive green-velvet-draped windows on each of the landings. Dated and fading slightly but wonderfully grand.

I like to arrive at the flat at least half an hour before my booking. I can just about do it in 15 minutes but it's a flap and I hate to be rushed. Opening the door to a client with an air of calm, poise and sophistication is tricky when two minutes previously you've been brushing your teeth while simultaneously making the bed and trying to find your other Jimmy Choo.

A Day in the Life of . . .

The first thing I do when I come in is turn on the heaters. There is one in the bedroom and one in the living room, and both go on full blast so it's really cosy when the client arrives. Then I prepare each room. The living room is spacious and bright but I always draw the curtains slightly to soften the light. Hides the wrinkles too! I put on a background CD on a low volume. Something easy listening. I boil the kettle (sometimes people want tea or coffee) and make a Rooibosh for myself. Yum.

Now I shower and retouch my make-up and make sure my hair is looking good. The make-up has to be perfect. I like to have smoky grey eyeshadow, long black lashes and fabulously glossy lips. Once I'm finished in the bathroom I pad around, wrapped in my pink towel and put all the clothes/bag/trainers and general crap I came with in a cupboard, out of sight, and prepare the bedroom.

The bed must have a clean white cover on the duvet and clean pillowcases. I fluff the pillows and smooth down the duvet so it's flat all over and perfectly positioned on the bed. There must be no hairs on the bed from a previous client so I do a 'hair inspection' to make sure.

On each side of the bed is a small white table. Out of the right-hand-side one I take out a packet of baby wipes (much better than tissues – they don't break up and get stuck all over the place), a singular nappy bag (for all used condoms etc), five condoms (two flavoured, one plain, one large and one 'trim'– well they couldn't call them 'small' could they!), a pot of non-scented massage lotion (non-scented is a good idea as reeking of 'orange and jasmine' when you normally smell of Hugo Boss could be a hard one for the client to explain), one bottle of lubrication (edible lube – yes you read that correctly, caramel and vanilla are the best), one packet of Wrigley's Extra thin ice and a couple of dildos – whichever ones take my fancy on the day. I also have a very nice orange butt plug which I bring out too, but this largely gets ignored as people don't seem to have a clue what it is.

In the bathroom I balance a fresh, folded towel (white) with a toothbrush on top, at the end of the bath. Everyone must shower and brush their teeth before they come anywhere near me. I think that's fair enough. Having 'just showered' isn't good enough. One man told me he was 'clean as a whistle', but after enquiring it transpired he'd had a shower that morning and it was well past 3 pm. Ahem. The toothbrush really is an absolute *must* as far as I'm concerned, and I send them back in if they try to skive!

On the left-hand-side table there are a couple of night-lights, a lighter and a couple of books. These I leave out at all times. Everything else is packed away. The books hopefully giving the impression I read at night – that I actually live there – This is mainly for the benefit of my landlady who I'm sure has a nosey round when I'm not there.

Now I get dressed. I love to wear a baby doll and killer heels or a fitted skirt and jacket suit. The one I have at the moment is *very* fitted and it's *very* sexy. Underneath, some hot underwear of my choosing – or perhaps something the client has specially requested. I love the 50s-style stuff right now and it suits my shape – I'm not a stick. Lastly some jewellery, a squirt of Chanel here and there and my Geena heels for a bit of sparkle. I don't want to look too formal. That's it. I'm done. All I have to do now is wait. I drink my tea and watch a bit of telly or read the paper if I have few minutes. At ten minutes before the booking time the client rings as I have instructed. I stress that they must call me exactly ten minutes before. No more, no less. If they call at 15 minutes to, which is rare, I get them to call back in five. They must follow my instructions exactly. It's my way of letting them know who's boss, if you will. Hell most guys *love* a woman in control. If they want to see me, they must play by my rules. It's also about respecting me, being courteous and listening to what I say. All of these things are important to me.

So the client calls from the station to get the address. I check the number is the same as the one he gave me when he booked and I take him through my security procedure. Before I give the address out I always let them know I have CCTV filming them coming into the building and that I employ a security guard for my own protection. Some people get a little freaked by this information but they still come – poor sods, if they were nervous before, now they are *really* nervous. That's good for me in a way. They feel more vulnerable. It's also a great client 'filter'. Anyone who is planning on robbing or attacking me will certainly think twice if they know they are being filmed or watched. People who are up to no good (and I've only come across one, thank fuck) do what they think they can get away with, and the way I try to set things up is to make sure people know they can't get away with anything. My intent is not to frighten people – well, maybe just a little . . . some people are wary of cameras – but on the whole, men realise that women have to protect themselves and cameras are no big deal these days. The whole of central London is on CCTV for God's sake!

When the client arrives I greet him with a kiss on the cheek and a big smile, invite him in and offer him a drink. It's always wine or water. Wine for the nervous and the more chilled-out client. Water people tend to be a little more uptight – maybe uptight is the wrong word but I sense that it can mean they are in bit of a hurry and just want to get on with things. Most people are pretty nervous unless they are 'seasoned punters', and the drinkers usually receive their poison of choice with much enthusiasm and a relieved smile.

While they are gulping down their wine, and starting on a second no doubt, I'm probably supping on a tea as usual and here the small talk starts. Out of an hour's booking I like to have about a ten-minute chat, more or less depending on the vibe you get from the client. Some people rabbit on for ages – this is definitely nerves and of course I will happily listen for as long as they like. Others down their drink quickly, refuse a second and sort of perch on the edge of the sofa expectantly. Most are happy to chitchat for ten and let me be in charge of the proceedings. I'm sure most guys are just quite happy you are the girl they saw in the ad and you can string a sentence together.

A Day in the Life of . . .

Okay so now it's shower time, for the client. Yippee. I always *tell* them that they are having a shower – in the nicest possible way of course. I never ask. That way they don't get a chance to refuse. I learnt that technique working in restaurants. They call it 'suggestive selling'. It's very crafty and I don't agree with being sneaky to get extra money out of people but God damn it's fabulous for getting people to wash!

I tell them exactly how to use my temperamental shower and inform them that there is a towel and a toothbrush there for them, and they have to use them both. Big grin. Then I shut the bathroom door and leave them to it. They can help themselves to anything, I tell them, which is basically an assortment of aftershaves, deodorants and breath fresheners. If they really want they can borrow my make-up too. This I say with a wink or something and this usually breaks the ice and gets a smile out of them if they are still utterly petrified.

While the client is crashing and banging around struggling with the shower I have a giggle to myself and then bring the CD player and drinks into the bedroom and select some sexy music. Aaliyah (RIP) is my favourite. All the songs are the perfect tempo for the bedroom – starting off slowly and then peaking and then ending quietly. Perfect for a booking. The mighty Brownstone another winner. If they are taking ages I might do some stretches or dance around a bit and prat around in front of the mirror, checking for spots or any new wrinkles that might have appeared in the night. When I hear them brushing their teeth I light the candles, and wait behind the bed-room door ready to open it as he emerges from his bathroom ordeal. I need to do this because on leaving the bathroom you are faced with 3 doors that all look exactly the same. I know which is which but Joe Bloggs doesn't, and if left to their own devices I might have them ending up on the landing and that could be tricky to explain to the neighbours. And so, eventually appears the dripping, towel clad, and usually slightly sheepish-look-ing client. I usher him in and note the large cloud of deodorant billowing out of the door behind him. Nice. Men do tend to overdo the deodorant thing. Again, nerves. Still, better to smell like they've been dipped in a vat of Lynx than BO any day.

I take their towel and put it on a radiator to dry and give them their drink. 'Make yourself at home,' I say, gesturing towards the bed. We drink, we talk for a moment and then I offer a massage. I do the back, shoulders and neck. I keep it short — about five minutes or so. I don't want to take the piss. Then I get them to turn over and I lie on top of them or by their side and ask them if they are feeling relaxed now. I look right into their face — we kiss and cud-dle, and I try to get a feel for what kind of sex they want. Some guys just lie there and want me to take the lead. Others are much more tactile and get quite passionate. I ask if they have anything particular that turns them on — try to get them to open up a bit. It's amazing how many peo-ple have never been asked that question. Mostly clients just want to please me, which was surprising at first. Hey

A Day in the Life of . . .

— I'm not complaining! If someone wants to make me come and then pay me for it that's fine by me.

I think they can see that I am quite happy to be there, out of choice not coercion, and at ease with my body and that makes a big difference to the client. I always find up until the point of nakedness, things are more stilted. There is less bullshit when you are naked for sure. I like *naked* and I like to mince around during a 'break' with just my dangerously high heels on, blabbing on about something or another while changing the CD or getting a drink. I probably look ridiculous, arse wiggling away and my hair askew but it's my place, it's my shout and I don't care. I'm having fun. Work can get terribly dull if there's no fun. It is what you make it. And who says being a whore can't be fun. Plus I like to entertain, I've discovered. I like to be funny but without losing the 'sexiness' of the moment. I personally think being funny is sexy but that's just me.

It's a bit like walking a tightrope of subtle behaviour traits. From the first phone contact I need to be 'professional' without being curt and 'easy-going' without sounding blasé. On meeting I need to be 'authoritative' without being bossy, 'witty' without being a smart arse, a 'good conversationalist' without being over-chatty and in the bedroom I need to look natural, sexy and at ease without looking like I've done this a million times.

I enjoy my chosen career. To some this may sound bizarre, of course it has its moments but it is never anything too drastic and I don't spend a ten-hour shift with my clients! I very much like the people I meet. They are polite, friendly men on the whole but make no mistake – they have been *rigorously* sifted before they get to me and by the time they are sitting on my sofa I'm 99 per cent sure I like them and that we'll get on. The people I see treat me infinitely better than when I was a nurse or when I waited on tables or when I worked in a shop. It hasn't put me off men and it hasn't put me off sex, but then I don't see that many clients, maybe one a day, and I have the luxury of being picky about who I see. Some people would see me as 'unfortunate' but for me it's quite the opposite. I feel very fortunate. I am my own boss, I can work or not work when I choose, I have lots of time to travel, I have hobbies, I see my friends, which in this day and age is pretty rare. I have a very decent disposable income and I am treated like a queen virtually every time I go to work. How many people can say that? I am lusted after, I am adored and I am complimented daily.

I see that what I do is, ultimately, about making people feel great, and I like that. Clients want to feel good. We all do. Maybe it is through the sex or maybe it's something you say to them. Of course it's about money and time and freedom from the rat race, but genuinely making people feel good about themselves is very rewarding and in my job I have the opportunity every day to really make someone's day, or make them feel more confident about their sexuality, or teach them something new, or give them a different perspective on their relationship problems, or tell them they have a great bum when they thought it was shit or whatever. I can't think of anything else I'd rather do right now.

A Day in the Life of . . .

Lyn's Story

Some weeks I can work like a demon, doing the rounds of several establishments. This week, for instance, I have been working lots as I worked for an escort agent last week and earned next to nothing! So making up for it this week, so far . . . I did a shift at the new brothel, one I want to start working at as it's very busy. It was Brisbane's first brothel, it's very hard to get shifts there as they have 45 girls on the books there and can only have five working at one time. So anyway, I did Tuesday night there 5 pm – 1 am; Thursday 4 pm – 12 am at Tigerlily, Brisbane's newest and most stylish brothel – they also charge a bit more, but it's not busy yet as it is only new; then went onto Purely Blue (the busy one) and did 1 am – 9 am, came home, slept three hours and went to Tigerlily 4 – 11 pm. I just got home now and start back at PB 9 am – 5 pm then Tigerlily 5 pm (it's meant to be 4 pm) until 12 am, so I am feeling bit knackered.

* * *

These are four individual's personal experiences of escorting. As you can see it can be both rewarding and harrowing. However escorting is not the only form of sex work.

Chapter Five

Other Forms of Sex Work

There are quite a few other ways to tap into men's desire to spend money in exchange for some kind of sexual fulfilment, and not all of them involve actually having sex with men. As with escorting, the amount of money you can make generally comes down to how good you are at what you do. Some 'jobs', like domination, require that you learn a lot and practise hard to hone what you do. Others, like text and phone sex, require very little other than a good imagination and a high boredom threshold. Some, like maiding and driving, are almost totally passive roles while others, like street prostitution and being an independent escort, need the individual to have a heightened awareness of, amongst other things, one's own safety.

Stripping

Stripping, lap dancing, pole dancing, erotic dancing – they are all pretty much the same thing in that they involve the tantalising exposure of the body for money. If you are young, beautiful, fit, a good dancer and a bit of an exhibitionist then stripping can be a great way to make money. In England, in the more established clubs, you generally audition for a job just as you would for an acting or modelling job. You need to look great. There is a huge amount of competition for places in reputable clubs so the fitter you are, the better you dance and the hornier your outfit at your audition the better chance you will have of getting in. Working in these places is just like any other 'straight' job. You are given specific shifts and are expected to turn up for them on time – girls who do not tend to get 'fined' by the establishment or lose their jobs quite quickly.

Most places have what they call a 'house mother'. She is the woman responsible for the girls. She is the person you telephone when you have a problem, she chooses your stage name, fixes your hem quickly at the last moment, sorts out any problems that might occur between girls, stops girls getting too drunk with the clients and generally takes care of everything backstage. In larger establishments you will generally perform on a stage. In Stringfellows, London's most famous venue, there are three girls on the stage at any one time. There is a pole in the middle of the stage and the girls rotate – ie your first dance is stage back left, your second is stage back right and then you go on to the pole. The slower and more seductive you can make this process the better. There are many places that now run stripping and pole dancing courses both in England and the USA. The most comprehensive list of these can be found at www.mypole.co.uk which has a huge list of schools and contacts in Britain, America and Europe. When you finish on the stage you then circulate around the club to find men who either want to sit and chat and drink with you or men who want you to dance privately for them. Both these things are chargeable. When the client arrives at the club and pays his entrance fee he is also able to 'purchase' the club's own 'money' with his credit card which is essentially paper vouchers with which he can purchase time, beauty and alcohol in the club.

> Most men don't bring in much cash and then they get drunk and carried away and get out the credit card.

In all large reputable clubs in England touching is not permitted, and there is generally quite heavy security on hand should any girl encounter a guy who gets a little out of control. Though this works both ways – if a girl is deemed to be getting too close to a client when dancing for him she may be reprimanded by the management or even 'fined'.

Your earnings tend to work like this. Customers will give you cash or paper vouchers they have bought from the club that represent money for you to dance for them. At the end of the evening you cash these in for real money, but the club will charge 'commission' for the 'transaction' and deduct a 'house fee' and any 'fines.' How the clubs get away with this is that not only do they charge the men to watch you they also charge the stripper what is called a 'house fee'. (The clubs also quite often charge the client a 'commission' to purchase their money and to redeem any of it back into real cash – should he not have spent it all.)

A good stripper with a sharp mind can make an awful lot of money, as Marilyn, a professional stripper, tells us:

> I tried a couple of places but ended up at Stringfellows, the poshest strip club going. I had a life, a love and the beginning of my career as an artist. I was looking for money and Stringfellows had plenty of it. Unbelievably I stayed for three years. Nothing competes with London's financial advisors not to mention the visiting Arabian sheiks. It was a matter of course to earn £500 a night and quite easy to make over a grand. The girls were stunning and they were cut-throat. A night could be ruined by a lack in confidence and you could walk away with nothing but your tears. This happened to us all from time to time. But in general I was a much better stripper. More in control of my body and mind.
>
> Despite my long respite in this chandelier-sparkling, leopard-printed 'gentleman's club' my time there is not marked by anything very memorable. There were scandals but they had nothing to do with me. The club's owner encouraged us to be his 'angels.' He prided himself on it being a clean club and rules were strict. Not to mention the fact that we were located in posh Westminster, he'd

lose his license. Touching was forbidden completely. We were a fully nude club but this was done discreetly. No spread eagles only butterflies.

What strikes me most about my time at Stringfellows was a sense of routine. Three years is a long time. The putting on of make-up, the costumes. The washing out of your thong. The waxing and shaving. The boredom of the incessant chatter in the dressing rooms. The tedious waiting around for customers to show up. The only distraction for me was the beauty of the girls, some of whom I could never tire of watching. Annie, who looked like a cross between Jessica Rabbit and Betty Page. Patti, who was our resident nymphet. We all watched each other and then we'd watch ourselves in the wall-to-wall mirrors. If I'm honest there was a thrill in that. There are not that many outlets in life for the kind of extreme sex appeal we got to express. We turned ourselves on. Girls aside, I suppose what was most memorable about the place was the money. That was when Stringfellows got exciting. It was the kind of place where you would do nothing but sit in VIP with some guy from Dubai for an hour and drink champagne. Then he'd signal for you to go and you would walk to the end of the bar and ask his white bodyguard for the money. Ask for any sum you wanted and you got it, no questions asked. After 11 September the club slowed down as expected.

Other Forms of Sex Work

Though things picked up eventually our Middle Eastern clients tapered off. By the time Tony Blair joined Bush in the Iraqi war, they'd all but stopped coming. Financially speaking, this was a tragedy.

Though they hid behind their astronomical bank accounts and upper-class mannerisms, the clientele in this club were as sad and pathetic as all men at strip clubs the world over. Still the club had a certain air. Celebrities would drop in, pop bands too. Women were welcome. This facade of respectability made it a reasonably pleasant place to work, but it was a facade. I don't know how many of the girls sidelined as prostitutes but there were plenty. I finally got the regular I felt I'd deserved in the form of Ronnie. He was CEO of a big bank that will go unnamed. He was harmless, rather sweet. But something about him was distinctly sad. He was in his thirties, reasonably attractive, married with children. We would spend hours together. He would only come there to see me. He would get drunk enough to fall down stairs. And he would never leave without paying me at least a grand. My biggest night with him was £1,900. It seemed to almost pain him to come in, but once there he was in freefall. I saw Ronnie at the club about three or four times a month for three quarters of a year. I'd always felt that eventually one of these frightfully rich men would decide that they liked me as a person and would want to become my patron and friend. I thought that maybe Ronnie could be the one. Ronnie and I had exchanged email addresses and he wrote to say he was coming to town on business and could he take me out. We had dinner and drinks. He was a gentleman, as always, but after that it was never the same. The magic of these relationships is your unavailability. Either that or your total and complete abandon. Don't ever believe the girls who say they don't have to fuck their sugar daddies. They're lying. Anyway Ronnie was big money for me for a time.

Other girls, it must be said, were much more committed, much more ruthless, and as a consequence much richer. I tended to work as little as necessary. Two days a week, maybe four at most. A lot of earnings went to my boyfriend. I was making so much money that the thought of him getting £40 for an eight-hour bar shift was ridiculous. We were living together and I wanted him around me all the time. At least in the beginning. So I ended up supporting two people for about two years in one of the most expensive cities in the world. Ladies, don't do what I did. It will end in resentment. Nonetheless we had a good standard of life. We ate out, went to movies and art shows. We travelled. I bought expensive face creams and occasionally splurged on £400 dresses. Most importantly we used the money I made to support our art. We did things no artists at the beginning of their careers would have been capable of through my sheer financial power. All in all my life outside the club was exciting, new and progressing towards a greater goal. If detachment is one key to surviving the business, purpose in life is another.

I've stopped dancing now. It came to an end at 28. That is a six-year span in the sex industry. The better portion of my twenties. Life has been a struggle since hanging up the stilettos. I've been out about a year. Luckily I am smart and I have options but it is really hard to come off the money and even more so the lifestyle. By lifestyle I mean the free time and the knowledge that you can pull yourself up out of the gutter in one night. But let's not romanticise. Stripping is hard work. The toll is physical, emotional and spiritual. If you get to 30 and all you have to say for yourself is that you are a stripper, you're in trouble. A gap in your resume that big is going to be hard to fill. You had better be sure you have something to show for your time and your money because you know what? You're not so pretty once the lights come on.

The other kind of stripping in England is done in pubs or 'gentlemen's bars', generally during the day. You dance and then you go around the crowd with a pint jar and collect whatever they give you. This can be demoralising, but, as Kirsty points out, no worse than some other jobs:

In Good Company

I tried door-to-door marketing – it's a bit like stripping but without taking your clothes off and with little chance of making any real money. At least when I was at Browns I always knew I would go home with something.

Stripping in America is quite a different issue, as Denise, who stripped in New Orleans prior to Hurricane Katrina, tells us:

Stripping in New Orleans is an institution. If you are a girl and you look good you'd be crazy not to do it. I started when I was 22. All my friends were strippers and all the guys we knew delivered pizza. Sometimes we'd have them deliver to the club. No one was shocked by anything. Customers in New Orleans come in about three stripes – sad locals, harmless tourists and convention men. New Orleans is a big convention town. In our dressing room we would have lists provided by the local business bureau saying things like April 3–7 IBM convention – 7,000. April 14–19 US Cattle Association – 4,000. That's 4,000 men away from their wives on corporate credit cards. Pay day. The way it works is you do a dance for 20 bucks. In New Orleans there is a fair share of wriggling on a customer's lap. But we kept our panties on. Things happened all the time though. It's the dirty south. If the customer wanted they could spend the hour in a VIP room for

Other Forms of Sex Work

$400–500. That's the way to make your money. Yeah things can get weird. You get drunk on endless champagne and I think almost everyone I knew got a bit carried away at times, myself included. No one ever lost sight of the money though.

One customer I had paid me $50 a dance, but he wanted me to wear these really ugly suntan pantyhose. Anyway it was kind of embarrassing to do in the main club area so I said if he wanted to go on with it we'd better get a private room. He was in ecstasy at the sight of these hose so off we went. After about 45 minutes of this tedious behaviour I asked him what was with the pantyhose? He said when he was a little kid he had a crush on his friend's mom. He used to go into her bathroom, open the hamper and get out her dirty hose. He would masturbate with them, of course. Pretty predictable so far. Then he says that one day the kid's mom walked in on him. He was mortified but instead of freaking out on him the lady tells him to keep going. From then on this became a regular event for the two of them all the way through high school. As I shimmied around in my suntan hose I thought to myself, well at least this guy has found an outlet for his fantasies. Otherwise he may have been out there in the streets becoming renowned as the pantyhose strangler.

People are fucked up and you find a lot of them in strip clubs. The men are sad and pathetic as a rule, even if it is not openly apparent behind their bravado boy's club bullshit. The girls have fun, a bit of guilt, a lot of insecurity (though this oscillates with the discovery of their own sex appeal) and a lot of money. Let me stress that New Orleans is a blast. Clubs are come and go as you please and stay open till 6 am. They are 24 hours during Mardi Gras. Occasionally you'd get some cute younger guys or a band from LA and the party would leave the club. Most nights me and Nina would ride our bikes home at about four in the morning, stop at the diner staffed entirely by queens, eat fluffy, buttery omelettes to soak up the champagne valleys in our stomach, and make it home by dawn with close to a thousand or more between us. New Orleans was so cheap that sometimes we'd go two weeks without working. Looking back, I did some pretty outrageous things and in the dirty world of one's private masturbatory life the spectres of New Orleans VIP rooms are the nasty bits of business that often come and visit me. What's the turn-on? My youth and beauty and the sheer filthiness of it all as far as I can tell. How do I feel about this? Well it ain't *Romeo and Juliet*.

Domination

Domination is tough. You need to be physically and mentally on the ball and you need to have a strong stomach.

Other Forms of Sex Work

Men who use professional dommes are predominantly, in my opinion, damaged. Bryan's story gives us an idea:

> I was in foster homes from the time I was six – no one wanted me. I started cutting myself when I was about 12. The only thing that stopped me was discovering tattooing and piercing, but when I got to my twenties that wasn't enough – I hated myself and my loathsome life. Then I found Mistress Nastasia; I go to see her whenever I can afford it and she beats the crap out of me and I feel better. I still cut myself if I can't afford to go see her.

Some girls like a playful spanking while sexually excited but the man who wants his genitals mutilated or tortured has, in my opinion, some kind of deep-rooted socio/sexual trauma – quite a lot of regular dominatrix clients admit to having been abused as children. Consequently these people need to be dealt with sensitively. If you are not the kind of person who can read beneath the psychological lines then domination is not for you.

A good dominatrix is trained in many skills, not just human psychology. She needs to know at least basic anatomy and first aid skills are a must. She must be able to cane or whip accurately, and, if required to, not mark the client, many of whom are married. She needs to be conversant with rope, chain, knots and human binding. She needs to know how to use electric probes, nipple clamps and piercing needles. She needs to know how to fuck a man with a strap-on. She needs to know and understand the mathematics and problematics of suspension – if you hang someone from the ceiling by his ankles you have to know how high to hoist him so that he does not crack his skull open. She needs to understand the principles of feminisation – forcing a man to appear and act as a woman. She also needs to fully comprehend sensual deprivation and its effect on the psyche and sexuality.

Many women come to domination because generally, apart from body worship (mostly this involves sitting on the client's face), there is no actual sex involved. This is supposed to be part of the 'power' trip, but the irony here is that the client dictates at the beginning of the session when he pays what it is that he requires – so although the role of dominatrix is the one of the all-powerful woman it is the man who actually dictates what happens in the session.

Most professional dungeons have at least a main chamber with all the tools and implements of the trade, a medical room where 'medical' procedures can be performed, a small dark room for locking people into, a full 'drag' wardrobe and a living area for the dominatrix and her 'maid' to relax in between clients. (The maid's job is also another way to make money in the sex industry – she answers the phones, buys the supplies and wine and generally looks after the dominatrix, the rates for a maid are generally a percentage of what the dominatrix makes.)

Most dommes dress up to the hilt in fetish gear – mostly leather and rubber as this heightens the fantasy element they are trying to create with and for their clients. The clothing and the equipment are not cheap so be sure before you invest lots of money in them that domination is what you really want to do. The best way to learn domination is to 'apprentice' yourself to an experienced working dominatrix. Or hit the fetish scene in your own city and get involved as Kathryn did.

> I was a natural submissive and I used to go to all these great clubs in the hope of getting someone to tie me up and whip me but because of the way I looked people assumed I was a dom. I ended up doing 'shows' at the clubs with another woman, Jennifer, where we would torture willing guys for the crowd. She got a job in a well-known dungeon. Then she got me a job there too. She taught me everything.

The best way to find out about events in your area is to go online – www.londonfetishscene.com is a great and comprehensive site for both the aficionado and the 'newbie' in England or http://bondage.com for the USA. Like everything else – do your research. The fetish scene can seem rather daunting and 'closed shop' at first entry, but persevere – some of them are really quite nice.

A good dominatrix should be unshockable and unshakable but it can be hard, as Margaret, a dominatrix in New York, found out when she first started:

> There were four dungeon rooms, a medical room, a consultation room and a lounge/office on the

In Good Company

28th floor of a non-descript office building in Chelsea. There was a daytime shift and a night-time shift. We were open noon to midnight. On each shift there were about four or five girls. In between consultations and sessions we'd smoke pot on the fire escape, watch horror movies and generally giggle our heads off. If only someone could have recorded our conversations. It was not unusual to make cameos in each others' sessions or to ride on our client's back out into the lounge, spurring them on by digging in our heels and having them polish everyone's boots with their tongue. Sometimes we'd just throw our food at them.

My very first training session was with a client named Nick. I walked in and this quite substantial black man was sat upon the black leather bondage table completely naked and frantically jerking off. My fellow dominatrix who was training me turned and said, 'This big gorilla wants you to tell him what a filthy nigger he is.' My mouth dropped. To call a black man a nigger is just not the done thing in my world. I had a moment of confusion and panic, but quickly realised this was his game. He was paying us $200 dollars an hour to have torrents of racial abuse hurled at him. To bend and beg and humiliate himself in front of us white women. I found the whole thing terribly traumatic on one hand but completely within reason on the other. After all in sexual situations how many self-respecting women like to be called dirty whores who are going to get what they deserve? Nonetheless I couldn't really get over my political correctness and Nick must have sensed this. He wouldn't become one of my regulars. He was, actually, a very lovely man who, once re-suited and booted, ceased to be a huffing, debased gorilla and became a charming, upwardly mobile African-American.

The psychosexual world of BDSM can be both fascinating and rewarding but it is by no means a casual thing, as Mistress Anna explains:

For starters, giving pleasure is the greatest source of power. By touching bodies, squeezing flesh, pressing buttons, and breaking skin, I guide him through his ordeal and assist in his pleasurable release. I get satisfaction out of lancing the blister and relieving the pressure. I can care about him for an hour and know nothing about him, and never see him again. I dress up in rubber and believe in my authority and wisdom. I trust my intuition, assert my influence, evolve a diatribe. I embody beauty and sexual power. And then I make him believe – because he came here to believe. Now that we both believe, we have a fantasy in action and a room full of tension and possibility. One hour to manipulate and make him feel what he doesn't usually feel. We'll vibrate between reality and fantasy, pain and pleasure, and all the opposites. It's a love pact between strangers that gets erased after an hour. I asked for a challenge and now it's stretched out naked on a rack in front of me. Who is he? What's he want? Where's his threshold? What's the magic word? There's a stranger at the door and his secret desire is about to be my responsibility. It's up to me to do something with it, make something of it, strike the right cord. It's just a game, simple and complex, perverted and benign. The man knows his place. Other treats include a captive and adoring audience, license to ramble, to pose, to experiment with words and minds, and intimidate with silence. At work today I sharpened my skills, strained to listen, tried to connect, and partook in his easy ecstasy. He was grateful. He paid me well. It was no more or less useful than, say, a concert in a vacuum, but it's a tender job with ample reward.

Domination, like escorting, is a sex industry service that can be financially rewarding and lucrative, and can be mentally rewarding if you find that your interaction with someone actually improves their quality of life. But it does have its drawbacks. If you are not strong enough psychologically in yourself it can find you experiencing your own emotional damage, as Laura, an American student in London, tells us:

Other Forms of Sex Work

My graduate studies took up a lot of my time, London costs a fortune and these facts meant the sex industry. I called round a bit and eventually ended up in a dungeon in Soho. It wasn't particularly posh. It was somewhat depressing in fact. It was located in the basement of one of London's typical rambling Georgian homes and could have done with a good scrub and some new equipment. There was just me and the 'maid', which is the term applied to the woman who answers the phones and makes appointments in such establishments. This title reeks of the British class system. My 'maid', called Courtney, soon became my best friend. Britishness abounded in other ways as well. Noticeably lacking was creativity in the clients. The public schoolboy caning scenario was deeply repetitive. Despite my efforts no one seemed to want to try new things.

I worked eight-hour shifts and much of the time was spent with just me and Courtney smoking spliffs waiting for punters to turn up. An average shift saw me making between £200–300. It never went past £800. To be honest, my abstract fascination with pleasure and pain, humiliation and restraint, was starting to wear off by the time I started working there. I found it rather boring by the end. My waning interest in this murky but mundane world was that this London dungeon, which the clients had been coming to for years, pulled you in psychologically. In any form of sex work it is a mistake to get emotionally involved. Detachment is key.

I worked as a dominatrix for about six months. There were highlights. Cross-dressing. One of my clients was just this enormous hulk and the sight of him in drag was frankly frightening. My favourite cross-dresser was Jason, a lamb of a man, who loved his wife and had a respectable career but could not resist the temptation to take his daring to the street. For instance he would visit on his lunch break, dress up for me and then make me insist on him wearing frilly little girl socks under his trousers on the tube ride back to work. The idea was that when he sat on the tube his trousers would inch up and he would be exposed. His daring increased over the course of our interactions and for our final session we had an excursion. We took a black cab down to Old Compton Street at the other end of Soho. I remember the way my black patent leather boots looked getting out of the cab. They were the only indication of my role in our outing. I waited for him in a pub while he went to the loo and put on a little skirt. He left his suit jacket, shirt, shoes and socks on. In a move that I found shockingly brave given his sweet and earnest temperament, he insisted on walking back to the dungeon alone. A good fifteen-minute stroll. I took a cab back and I remember driving past him as he walked up the street, determined, sweating and frankly precious.

Other Forms of Sex Work

I can be quite sentimental and I supposed that in some way I'd helped him come to this strange victory.

There was also Michael. A pseudonym I later found out. Michael is a deeply damaged individual who has spent time in mental wards. He is also a brilliant thinker, a bit occult in his wanderings, but completely fascinating. In addition I discovered that he was an amazing photographer, though he hasn't picked up a camera since he fell apart. He was around 30 when we met. Our first session was conducted in the standard domme/sub way, but I quickly realised this was all too much for him. We simply talked after that. Mostly philosophy and art. He came religiously every week. Once he performed an exorcism on the dungeon, which was most likely the right thing to do. We eventually became friends. I decided that I could no longer take his money. Courtney and I realised he was an incredibly special human who had found his way to us out of sheer loneliness. I decided to see him outside the dungeon. He is very hard to spend time with because he is racked in so many ways by his paranoia, his stuttering and his episodes, but I have tried my best to be part of his life in small doses. Four years later we are still in touch. I see him about twice a year.

The final straw eventually came. This individual began calling about two weeks prior to his visit. He was coming from out of town and was making a really big production of it. He turned out to be in his seventies, speaking, dressing and acting like an MP. A very dirty vile one. A product of public schools and the perversions of old Britain. He brought me flowers and tried to act the gentleman, but it is very apparent when a sub is really masking a dom. In fact it always struck me as odd that though one is meant to dominate one is actually being told what to do and finds oneself doing it for money. It is truly a farce. At any rate the man was a bastard. At every turn he tried to correct me, telling me what to do. He was, strictly speaking, not behaving. He had booked a two-hour session and five minutes into it I knew this was going to be interminable. He wanted everything. Humiliation, beating, electrics, water sports, and, my fucking favourite, anal play. As a rule I avoided shoving dildos up men's backsides. It is quite enough to be exposed to their fat, disgusting, naked bodies. Sometimes it was unavoidable. Men who insisted were always told they must give themselves an enema beforehand. We are now getting into the realms of the truly gross. He began to infuriate me rapidly. I wanted to hurt him. Badly. But no matter what I inflicted on him his eyes burned and he cried for more. I was losing control of the situation utterly. By the time we got to the electrics I had them on full strength, a first for me, and I felt like an administrator of torture at the inquisition, except it wasn't working. I imagined him a master of the world. An evil gloating power baron who must be destroyed. I wanted to rape him and make his asshole bleed. When I pulled the biggest dildo I had in my arsenal from his arse it was covered in his excrement. I ran into the corner of the dungeon, as far away from him as I could possibly get, and gagged repeatedly. I screamed for Courtney, who came running, and told her to get this monster away from me. He was gleefully licking his own shit. I escaped into the office and screamed bloody murder. He was evacuated from the premises as soon as possible. It was my very last session as a dominatrix.

I soon went back to working in the 'real' world and it felt like a walk in the park. In a very short time the activities I'd been party to in the dungeon became unimaginable. Though I was always myself during the entire experience the person who could do what I did felt almost unknowable. Scarring? Well maybe that last session, but in general? No. More truthfully it all just seemed way beyond the call of duty. Despite the fact it had been my bread and butter, now you could not pay me to do it.

So, think very carefully about your own limits and desires before embarking on domination as a career.

Submission

The flipside of the coin to domination is of course submission. Allowing someone to dominate you for money. As with escorting, know exactly what you will and won't do beforehand and be honest about it.

The types of actual work a submissive can get are quite varied but all generally involve pain, so be very aware of what you are doing and what you really want before embarking on this as a genuine form of work. Many submissives work one week on and two weeks off in order for the bruises and cuts to heal. A popular form of this work in the UK is spanking parties where any number of women will circulate in a room of men and allow themselves to be spanked at will. The rates for this vary – I was once offered £150 for a three-hour afternoon session, which, needless to say, I turned down, and on another occasion £500 for two hours. If you like being spanked it can be fun but be prepared for your butt to be unusable for a few days!

As with domination before embarking on submission as a career I would strongly suggest getting out on the fetish scene in your own area first. Discover what it is in your own psyche that needs to be fulfilled. Here too you may actually meet working dommes who may be prepared to use you in their working dungeons, but be very careful – trust no one straight away, keep your eyes and ears open, and do not cloud your brain with drugs and alcohol – games sometimes go too far, submissive women can end up very badly hurt both physically and mentally, as Petra's story shows.

Other Forms of Sex Work

I had tried working as an escort but I didn't like it. The agency I worked for had an office above a dungeon and I used to hang out with the women who worked there. One day I was asked to be part of a scenario for which I would get £50. I was skint and I thought I quite liked the idea of being a little sex-slave girl so I said yes. We went into the chamber and the client seemed really nice. The Mistress tied him up in the middle of the room then she forced me to my knees, between his legs while tying my hands behind my back. When she forced my face into his cock and started screaming at me to bite it off I started to get really scared – I didn't know what to do. I begged her not to make me do it, the guy was whimpering but obviously loving every minute. I just wanted out. She called me an impertinent little slut and hit me across the back with her whip. By this time I was in tears but I stuck the session out – it got worse but I don't want to think about it. As soon as the session was over I got out of there and I never went back.

In New York working submissives in dungeons are much more common than they are in London and for some it can be a thrill, as Jordan shows:

I worked in a dungeon where we also did sessions as submissives. Whether or not you did this was a personal choice. I was never a domme's domme. I found the experience of hurting people and humiliating them abstractly interesting, but it was never a turn-on. Being a sub was. This could be dangerous work, but our dungeon had thin walls and several safety measures in place. If one of these guys really hurt one of our girls they would never have made it out the door and they knew it. But one did get bruises. I didn't like the pain so much. I guess I liked the humiliation and the tingle of fear. I'm one of those girls who like to be called a whore. Go figure?

I had a favourite client who I'd sub for. I can't remember his name. He was sort of short but good looking in a watered down Hollywood-actor way. He had issues. Sessions with him were pleasantly creepy. He'd stand me in front of a mirror and pull back the corners of my mouth. Through this grimace I'd have to say that I was a dirty girl, a whore and various other nasties. Look in the mirror and try it on yourself. Scary stuff. I'll never forget the first time he pulled my dress up over my head. It was black but it was spandex. He never knew that I could see him through the fabric. At least I don't think he did. I imagine what I must have looked like. Stilettos, skimpy thong, the features of my face standing out against the tight material, my hands above my head in cuffs attached to the ceiling. Suddenly he took the pose of a boxer. He did a little dancing in place. Then out flew his fists. Jab, jab, undercut. Each strike stopped just before it made contact with my breasts. I had to suppress a laugh despite being strangely turned on and mildly terrified. This guy was straight out of *American Psycho*, but apparently so was I.

Like domination, please think very carefully about your own state of mind and motivation for doing it before taking on submission as a viable form of work.

Text and Phone Sex

Phone and text sex are the easiest form of sex industry work there is, primarily because there is no actual face-to-face interaction with the client. However, overexposure to it can cause brain damage and a serious dislike of all men. Generally this is because the men who use these services are those with the basest level of sexuality. These are the men who cannot use prostitutes or escorts either because their communication skills are lacking or they simply don't have the wherewithal. The irony of this is that text and phone sex is the biggest con within the industry and for what the punter is actually getting can be inordinately expensive. In England the going rate for SMS (or text) sex is about £1.50 a message, for phone sex it is 10p–£1.50 per call.[1] In America and Canada all 1-900 (US and Canadian sex-line prefix number) calls cost $2.99–$5.99 a minute, usually with a $4.99 connection fee.[2]

In Good Company

As a text or phone sex operative you can work either from an office generating the messages or calls through a computer or you can work from home using your own phone line, depending on the company you work for. You will either be paid by the hour or by the message. Essentially, the operative feeds the fantasies of the client. You are writing or speaking basic porn with the object of getting the client off sexually (but not too quickly if your wage is paid by the message or call). This can be easy work particularly for those who are tied down to being in the home, ie single mothers, but can have its drawbacks, as Aileen shows us:

> I worked as a text sex operative for two years. I earned £5 per hour plus 3p commission on every text. In the beginning it seemed like a bit of a laugh, I mean these guys talk the grossest sex you can imagine – it would not turn any real woman on. There were guys who would literally text for hours about how they were going to fuck you so hard you would bleed, there was the guy who went on and on about you wanking him off with your gloves – I called him 'The Glove Fucker', there were ones who wanted to slit your throat at the moment of orgasm and, most disturbingly, ones who said they wanted you to be a young girl and those who 'confessed' to real or imaginary sexual contact with children. How they afforded it I'll never know. After a few months I found that I was

losing interest in sex and every man I met I would wonder if he was one of these guys. It just gets under your skin – I accept that many of them probably never had sex before and that was why their fantasies were so disturbing and cruel towards women.

Glamour Modelling

Glamour modelling, whether it be magazines (top shelf, obviously), newspapers (page three), television (satellite cable stations only) or on the web can be fun, but it is not terribly lucrative for most women and you do not have a choice with regard to exposure. Only embark on this course if you are not worried about who is going to see your face, or the rest of your body for that matter.

If you have a desire to appear in 'men's magazines', the best way to go about getting into them is to go along to your nearest purveyor of top-shelf magazines, purchase a few and look through them. Nearly all of them have a section asking for submissions from potential models. Get a friend or partner to take a few shots in the same vein, though not quite as explicit (don't give too much away before they have paid you something) and send them in. The publishers will do one of two things. They will either print the pictures you have sent and pay you anything between £10–50 per shot depending on the quality, sexiness and where they place the pictures, or, particularly if you have sent a covering letter explaining your desire to be a glamour model, they may forward your images to any of their house or freelance photographers who may then approach you for a proper shoot. The first course of action can be quite a laugh and can spice up your own sex life somewhat, as Anne and Tony found out.

> Tony and I started getting into taking sexy pictures of each other as part of our sex play. Just for a laugh we sent a few into one of the main porn magazines. They got printed and we loved it! Soon we were photographing each other every week and sending it off. The money wasn't great but we had loads of fun!

If you want to try approaching it from a more serious angle then get yourself a portfolio of professional shots for your own collection before approaching the newspapers and magazines. Be aware that they will want to see your face and, in the case of the magazines, will probably want to see shots of your genitals. While in England it is illegal for publishers to print a picture of a man with an erection penetrating anything, or for that matter a woman penetrating herself with anything, it is quite acceptable to print extreme close-ups of a spread vagina. If they like what they see they will generally arrange for you to meet and work with one of their house photographers.

In my experience most of these photographers tend to veer towards the very sleazy but one or two are genuinely okay and one or two are even women. Like every other form of work, turn up on time if not earlier and be well prepared with several changes of outfit, your make-up and a few accessories (take your own vibrator!). Most magazine shoots involve a 'story', which will require you to move through the stages of undress till you and the photographer get to the 'lips' shot. You will generally be asked to sign a 'model release form' which means that you have no rights over the images and they can use them wherever and as often as they like. A good going rate for a full shoot in London should be around the £200 mark but many photographers pay a lot less. So really, this is something to do more because you enjoy posing and exhibitionism than for the cash, as Charlotte explains:

> I love posing in sexy gear and I love having my photograph taken – it's when I am in my element. I tried stripping but I couldn't handle the guys so I had a go at glamour modelling. It is so much fun if you get a decent photographer, but I have encountered some guys who wanted to fuck me as part of the shoot – I always walk away from them, that isn't why I'm there. I'm a natural 34D so I do get quite a bit of work but you have to slow down sometimes or your face gets too well known and the magazines stop using your pictures because they feel you have been overexposed.

If you choose to go for modelling jobs on the web please be very aware of how universal it is and the fact that pretty much anyone can download your image and use it in any way that they want to. There are, like escort agencies, literally hundreds of glamour model agencies and, as with escorting, do your research and do not be coerced into doing anything you do not really want to do. Also remember that the word 'model' is quite often used as a euphemism for escort, so clarify what you will be expected to do before you do it. The best jobs to go for are the ones where the client has to register and 'pay per view' as this slightly minimises the amount of people who will access your image. Do not underestimate how many people access internet porn. Pornography on the net is big business. In 2001:

> there were 74,000 adult websites, two per cent of all sites on the web. It has been estimated that, each day since then, 20,000 new porn pages have been added. They generate profits of more than 1 billion dollars a year, which are expected to rise to some 5 billion dollars a year by 2005. For some, the use of those sites is compulsive. Perhaps one per cent of the visitors to sex sites, some 200,000, are 'cybersex compulsive'. That is the definition of people who spend more than 11 hours a week visiting sexually orientated areas.[3]

So be prepared for the backlash should anyone, like your dad, see it.

Other Forms of Sex Work

Porn

Porn films, unlike most of the other subjects in this chapter, do require sexual interaction. For women, getting into porn films is really quite easy primarily because so many people want to make them. Bear in mind that once you have done this there is no going back. A movie exists forever. You will generally be required to have undergone a three month AIDS/STI test to prove you are free from HIV and other sexually transmitted diseases, as most porn makers these days do not want actors wearing condoms. You will generally be required to be able to masturbate yourself and others on film, have sex with both genders and toys and do anal. Lots of anal. The porn industry is obsessed with it. If all this sounds good to you then approach porn makers with your portfolio. You may be required to do a 'test shoot', which means performing, quite often with the director or producer, for a run through to see whether you both look good on film and can perform sexually without inhibitions.

Some women like Jenna Jameson have found working in porn works for them. According to askmen.com:

> Jenna Jameson began her career as an adult film star in 1993. By 1996, the woman who had taken her stage name from a phone book had become a star, earning the triple crown of the porn industry: the XRCO Best New Starlet, The AVN Best New Starlet and the FOXE Video Vixen. She was the first entertainer to have won all three awards.[4]

In Good Company

Essentially, if you are going to enter the porn industry make sure you are making the right kind of money for what you are doing. Getting a couple of hundred pounds or dollars for committing yourself to celluloid is not necessarily such a great idea, as Jan found out:

> I gradually extended my comfort barriers to the point where I fucked some guy in his fifties in front of two to three other sweaty perverts to make a porno. I wouldn't do it again, well not in that set-up anyway.

Maiding

Maid is the term for the person, generally female, who works in brothels or dungeons opening the door, greeting and seating the clients and taking their money. In a brothel she ideally keeps an eye on the woman or women she is working with, changes sheets and buys in supplies like condoms. Although the 'maid' does not participate in sexual activity per se she can be arrested and charged with running a brothel because there is more than one person on the premises at a time. If she works in a dungeon she is required to clean before and after each session, take bookings for her dominatrix, facilitate the entry and exit of clients and take their money.

Most maids are paid a percentage of the earnings of the women they work for. It can be fun but it can be a thankless task, as Jess, who works in a central London dungeon, points out:

Other Forms of Sex Work

I have worked for Madame for about a year. I work three days a week and another maid does the other three. My first job is to check that the card boys have posted her cards up round the local telephone boxes. Then I go unlock the dungeon and clean up any debris from the day before. I thoroughly clean and sterilise the dungeon and the bath and medical rooms. The phone goes pretty constantly at this time of the day and I make appointments for all genuine clients. When Madame arrives I make her coffee, get her breakfast if she requires it and help her get dressed. Then we sit around and wait for the clients. When they arrive I check them out on the CCTV camera to make sure they do not look like police or trouble, then I let them in. I take them to the dungeon or the waiting room and inform Madame that they are ready and waiting. Madame has a small five-minute 'consultation' with them and comes back to me with the money, which I then lock away. Sometimes the clients like to be paraded around in front of me dressed up as naughty schoolgirls or human ponies. Sometimes they want a third person involved in their scenarios. On these occasions I will laugh and humiliate them if that's what is required or go into the dungeon and help Madame torture them. Sometimes they want me to play the submissive. I don't like this though – it feels too much like they have some kind of power over me personally. Though sometimes they will tip me for this. Most of the men are playing some kind of absurd psycho game that I find a bit disturbing – I can listen to their screams through the walls quite happily but I don't especially like being in the same room as them. That's why I'm the maid and she is the dominatrix. A lot of clients book appointments and then get cold feet and don't show so some days we can just be sitting around for hours on end. Madame gets bored very easily so I will roll her joints and buy her wine and try to keep her amused. It's the cash at the end of the day that makes it all worthwhile. I never leave with less than £40 – often it is more like £100. And when she is in session I get to do my own things.

Driving/Security

This job is generally done by men. They receive a percentage of the woman's money for driving them to outcalls, waiting for them while they see the client and then driving them home or to the next job afterwards. Some agencies use them in order to keep an eye on the girls both for the woman's security and to ensure the agency gets its money. For some women they are an essential, particularly in Australia where clients have a reputation for being quite aggressive. Nick worked as a driver up and down the Gold Coast of Queensland and New South Wales in Australia:

Mostly I work for one house near the Queensland/New South Wales border. Seven o'clock in the evening is when the action begins. Anything up to a dozen or 16 girls will arrive and go into a room to put their make-up on and do their hair, etc, then they go sit in a larger lounge with sofas everywhere. Some will remain in the house all night, while others do outcalls in cars like mine. You might ask where all these girls come from – well, some of them are from Sydney or Melbourne, up here for the sunny weather during the day and to make money at night. Others are down from Brisbane for the weekend on the pretext that they work at Gold Coast hotels as night receptionists, etc. Well, that's what they tell their families and friends.

One Friday night an attractive brunette, Zoe, arrived from Brisbane and stayed in the house till Sunday morning. Her husband back in Brisbane thinks she is working in a hotel. Unfortunately for her, her husband's best friend walks into the house out of the blue. Talk about being in the wrong place at the wrong time! They are both surprised and she takes him aside for a chat. Knowing him very well and, obviously, not wanting her husband to find out what she is doing, she has to come to some kind of agreement with him. You could say he blackmailed her. Eventually she agreed to meet with him once a week in their hometown of Brisbane, he would pay her just like in the Gold Coast brothel but she had to do it unprotected. Talk about a catch-22 situation! She didn't want to lose her husband, who, incidentally, detested the sex industry, but she was also working to pay her husband's court fines and keep him out of jail. Some women pick them!

Independent Escort

I would not advise any woman to go straight into the sex industry on her own, but if after working with a reputable agency you feel that you have developed the knowledge and strength to branch out independently, here are the necessary steps to take. From the outset be prepared to have to cover your own costs for a while. Going independent is a business decision and a bit of a gamble but with determination, perseverance and some well invested cash it can be very lucrative and rewarding.

The first thing you need is somewhere to work from. You could either find a flat of your own or go in with other girls who are like-minded. Both options have advantages and disadvantages. In England women who work together, ie from the same premises, face the danger of being charged with brothel-keeping, although it can make you feel safer and, of course, splits the rent. Or you could of course rent a cheap hotel room.

Next is the ever-present mobile phone.

Now all you have to do is advertise yourself. You will need your own website. As has been previously stated about agencies and photographers, the same also applies to sex industry website builders and promoters – check around, do your research, find out what the current rates are for the kind of site you require and watch out for shysters, conmen and rip-off merchants. (As with agents and photographers, there are many more women website builders and designers than there were a few years ago.) The internet has several good sites for independents to join. The best in my opinion are Executive Escorts (www. executive-escorts.com) and Cherry Girls (www.cherry-girls. co.uk), but try a few. Exchange banners with as many other adult websites as you can. Advertise yourself on the daily sex message boards, invest in local newspaper advertising and advertising on sites like Eros (www. eros.com) and get your regular clients to write reviews on you.

Always run a security check on any client who you have not seen before. If you are visiting his home get his full name, his address, his landline number and who that land-line is registered to, then ring directory enquires. If he doesn't check out you don't go. If he is in a hotel simply ring reception and ask if he has checked in yet. If he is not who he says he is, you don't go. If he is coming to visit you, do not give him the address until he is five minutes away from the location. When he arrives let him know that your 'driver' is just out on the street and is moments away should you need him (whether this is true or not). If you have a friend who can clock-watch for you, give them the details of who you are seeing, where you are going and your expected times. Phone them before and after the booking so that they know that you are okay. Above all, be safe. Listen to your instincts. Don't do *anything* you don't want to do. Lara's story is typical:

> Almost all women coming into the industry will start off with agencies (and many very happily remain so) as you really need to be in the industry a while to get yourself up and running independently and to find out the best people to build sites, advertise, etc and do all the things that an agent does for you. As your confidence grows and you want to establish yourself more, it seems natural to want to do your own thing.
>
> It seems I was not dissimilar to others who had been working for a while and felt comfortable in the industry and who had also come to the realisation that it was far better to be working independently. The hope was that financially I would be better off, more in control and happier in my work. Yes, I would be taking a chance that my own advertising would bring in the same amount of work as being with an agent, but I felt prepared enough to take that risk rather than continue to pay 30 per cent of what I earn to the agent. Plus, from a marketing point of view, it seemed that a good deal of clients preferred independent women – having your own site conveys the message: I am organised and professional, I have my wits about me and, above all, that most probably you actually want to be in the

business. Visually, I could also have complete control over how I represented myself on the net, and that is perhaps the most important part of how you market yourself and in my experience greatly determines the type of clientele you receive. I took heed and took the plunge.

In the months since making the transition I have felt happier and more in control. I could speak to and evaluate each client personally, and didn't have to clock in and out with the agents daily. I am running my own business and I haven't looked back.

Street Work

I have left this section till last because I really did not want to include it at all, as to my mind it is not a viable form of sex work. The bottom line with street work is *do not do it!* Street prostitutes end up dead. Respect yourself and don't even contemplate this as a valid way to make a living. Whatever your situation, there should always be a better option than this. In a recent US study of almost 2,000 prostitutes followed over a 30-year period, 'by far the most common causes of death were homicide, suicide, drug- and alcohol-related problems, HIV infection and accidents — in that order. The homicide rate among active female prostitutes was 17 times higher than that of the age-matched general female population.'[5] In England, according to documentary maker Maggie O'Kane: 'In the past 10 years, at least 60 prostitutes have been murdered in the UK. Many more are missing.'[6]

Go to any street in any red light area in any city and watch the women working there – predominantly they are the disaffected, the physically abused, the drug addicted, the beaten. Do not allow yourself to become one of them because the road out is so hard it is more often than not impossible.

There are various resources at the end of this book for women in this situation. If you are one of those women and you are reading this now, please use them – have respect for yourself and do not allow men or life to use or abuse you. Please move on, there are other choices. You have but one life and one body – value it!

Chapter Six

The Media and the Law

The media and the law are the two things existing outside of the sex industry that impact on us mercilessly. While we have to live with them, a healthy wariness of the first and a working knowledge of the latter is only sensible.

The Media

In the UK the media's attitude to prostitution, sex work and women in general is that somehow everything is the woman's fault. Look at the recent exposure of the young famous football star who'd been 'caught' visiting a much older prostitute. While some papers did vilify the young man in question, most focused on 'the dirty old slag whore' who had trapped poor 'Mr Too Much Money Young Football Star' into her web of vice. If only life were that simple! Despite having a well-publicised romance with a gorgeous young woman this adult man felt the need to seek out the services of a sex worker. He was not dragged there kicking and screaming, he sought it out for himself. In the society we live in it is far easier to make sex appear as smut and turn the everyday into salacious disgust and outrage.

Look too at the recent publication of an anonymous escort's story where many male reviewers and journalists posited the idea that it couldn't have genuinely been written by an escort because the writing was too well educated for a 'working girl'. I also spoke with men at the time who did not believe that a woman could possibly have written it! Just for the record – many sex workers I know have either achieved degrees or are studying for one.

Bearing in mind that your average member of the public's exposure to the sex industry comes from the newspapers, which are informatively suspect; television, which over-glamorises some aspects of the industry while, with negative consequences, not providing enough accurate information; and phone box cards, the traditional form of advertising for girls working from flats, it is no wonder that your average person sees us as a blight to be removed from the visible face of society. This is why politicians and public figures periodically forward the idea of creating 'Prostitution Red Light Zones', which in my opinion would only ghettoise and alienate sex workers from society even more.

In my own experience in the sex industry, the pompos-ity of the generic male media as it condemns that which it consistently uses – both for 'sexxxsational' stories as well as those individuals who actually use the services of sex workers – has led me in the past to deny interviews to any but sympathetic women journalists writing for publications within the sex industry itself.[1]

The self-imposed morality crusade that many journalists and publications believe is 'what the public wants' has led on too many occasions to sex workers' stories and quotes being manipulated negatively by both the tabloids and the more 'serious' broadsheets, as Beverley, a working dominatrix and writer on women's sex issues, found out:

> LL came to interview me for some book project. I forget what the title was exactly – something to do with women who like porn or women who like SM. Maybe it was women who actually believe they have clits. Anyway, she came round to my flat and we talked for a while. I thought her questions were daft but I was too polite to tell her that, and I was still a bit pleased, generally, to be interviewed. So I wasn't being all that careful, and when it somehow came up in conversation I freely told her that I was adopted as a very young baby. Some time later, about three different people drew my attention to that day's *Guardian* newspaper, where LL was banging on in print about all these mad weird women, and what she said about me suggested that my interest in SM was because of 'the parents who abandoned her so long ago'. She didn't actually give any context, didn't mention adoption . . . and used a very thinly disguised version of my real name, hence my mates working out who she meant. Not only is her theory

the usual crap you got in those days (when women liking sex at all was pretty suspect) and still sometimes get, but the implied insult to my family – ie my mum and dad who adopted me and who are, in my book, my parents (never mind the biological bit) – still makes me furious.

Subsequent forays into the media just made me more cautious: you have to be very sure of yourself and never give them an inch – or, if you're going to be misrepresented make sure you're getting very well paid for it.

Television too plays its part in mythologising and misinterpreting the sex industry. We see docu-dramas about women working the streets with potentially devastating implications for the women who allow themselves to be filmed. This was highlighted by a recent BBC documentary series showing the face of a 'maid' in Soho handling the cash from jobs – allegedly a maid was attacked at knife point for the money just days after the screening of this show. We see whole programming series on pornography and porn stars, we have chat shows morning, noon and night where audiences tut or yell disapprovingly at any woman who admits to exchanging sex for cash or goods and we get the endless televisual fodder of 'improve your image, life and sexuality' reality television. Even when 'serious' investigative journalism is employed in television, I still believe that predominantly only the aspects that the producer, writer or broadcaster want you to see are employed. As ever this creates a biased and often hackneyed view of the subject, further disallowing the general public from adequately assessing the true reality of a situation. Yes, sex work has its victims and its abuses, however not all those victims are women and not all of the abuse happens all of the time to all of the women who work in the industry. Question everything you see. If society could think for itself it wouldn't need the kind of media we have today.

We have discussed entrapment previously and will go into it in more detail in the next section, but be very aware that journalists are just as capable as the police are – if not more so because their motivation is cash – of posing as clients or other working girls to get a story.

It is a good thing to keep abreast of media and public attitudes to the work we do but remember that not everything we see, hear or read is necessarily true. And as Jean Paul, a freelance tabloid journalist, freely admits:

> It's not about art; it's not about justice. It's not about the moral consequences of the story for those involved, it's all about cash. The more famous the target, the more salacious or sleazy the angle, the bigger the pay cheque. Sex sells, but sleazy sex sells more.

This is not to say that the media cannot be used positively, as the English Collective of Prostitutes (ECP) has done on many occasions:

> Since 1975 we have been campaigning for the abolition of the prostitution laws which criminalise sex workers

and their families, and for economic alternatives and higher benefits and wages so that no woman, child or man is forced by poverty or violence into sex with anyone. We provide information, help and support to individual prostitute women and others who are concerned with sex workers' human, civil, legal and economic rights.[2]

The Law

The information in this section is intended only to give an overview of the law on escorting and prostitution in various countries. It is not intended to be comprehensive. Please contact prostitute support groups or women's advice centres in your own country, many of which are listed in the resources section at the end of the book, to find out your exact legal position.

UK

The laws on prostitution vary throughout the UK; Scotland and Northern Ireland both have slightly different laws in place to England and Wales, so please check out your local position on prostitution.

In England and Wales, according to The Bar Council of the UK:

The Sexual Offences Act 2003 defines a prostitute as, 'a person (A) who, on at least one occasion and whether or not compelled to do so, offers or provides sexual services to another person in return for payment or a promise of payment to A or a third person.'[3]

As mentioned in Chapter One, escorting in England and Wales is legally different from prostitution in that what you and your agency are selling is your time. What you do in that time is strictly between two consenting adults. However most agencies are, in truth, actually controlling prostitution for gain.

Ian from SW5 says:

> The law for escorts is really really simple – they can both say, 'I'll have sex with you for money' and do it. It's the people running the agencies and brothels and those people doing street work who have problems . . .

SW5 is an organisation working with men and transgender people who sell sex. Its website provides excellent legal information. They have very kindly allowed me to quote from their web pages throughout this section.[4] They say,

> It is legal to work for escort agencies, whether or not you are offering sexual services . . . Escort agencies where the staff are only providing 'social escort' services, rather than sexual services, are legal.

However, many, if not most, escort agencies are there to provide sexual services. SW5 believes that:

In Good Company

What stops . . . the agencies . . . being raided and closed down is that agencies tend to be much lower down the list of police priorities than street work or brothels.

However if the police do decide to take an interest in you, they have repeatedly demonstrated they are quite prepared to pose as clients and potential workers in order to prove you know what's really going on, despite disclaimers like 'Any fees paid to our escorts are for time and companionship only and anything else that may occur is a matter of personal choice between two consenting adults only'.

We discussed entrapment in Chapter Three and, should the police take an interest in you, the best way not to get into trouble is to make sure that you never accept cash or talk about exchanging cash for sex with more than one person present at any time.

Section 53 of the Sexual Offences Act covers 'controlling prostitution for gain', and includes, for example, telling an escort where to go to meet a client. Agencies also have to be wary of section 52 of the Sexual Offences Act 2003, which says 'causing or inciting prostitution for gain' covers encouraging someone to become a prostitute in the expectation that you or anyone else will gain as a result. SW5 also say:

This . . . is likely to include saying things such as 'no experience required' when advertising for new staff.

It's okay (under this clause anyway) to employ someone who's already a prostitute – ie someone who's ever
given or offered any sexual service for money – but
employing someone who says they have never done so
is very risky . . .

Niki Adams from ECP says:

This may become one of those myths where people
say it's okay to hire women who have a record but not
someone who doesn't. No cases have turned on this
point. In practice the opposite takes place and agency
bosses are charged under all kinds of circumstances.
Conviction depends on how good legal representation
is and whether women give evidence against him/her.[5]

Though as Ian from SW5 points out:

It's not a record (ie a conviction) that's the defence,
it's being a 'prostitute' already. And that's staggeringly
easy (offer to kiss someone for a million pounds and
you're one too!).

SW5 say:

It is unlikely that agencies who are employing adults
who have clearly made an entirely voluntary choice to
do the work will be charged with 'trafficking within
the UK for sexual exploitation', . . . section 56 of the

Sexual Offences Act 2003, which prohibits 'arranging or facilitating the movement of someone when intending to do or facilitate anything which if done would involve the commission of an offence', . . . but if the agency is being prosecuted for 'controlling prostitution for gain' and has helped staff move around (for example by booking taxis for them or having drivers take escorts to bookings) then it is a possibility.

SW5 also state:

It is not illegal to advertise sexual services, although if the ads are extremely graphic and are likely to 'deprave or corrupt' persons likely to see them, they may fall foul of the Obscene Publications Act 1959. Also, it's illegal under the Criminal Justice and Police Act 2001, and it applies to any public phone anywhere, except where U18s aren't allowed.

It is an offence for a person to keep, or to manage, or act or assist in the management of a brothel. According to SW5 the law defines a brothel as:

Any premises – including private flats, saunas, massage parlours – will be classed as a brothel if they are used by *more than one* man or woman for 'physical acts of indecency for . . . sexual gratification', whether on the same day or on different days – 'in series or in tandem'. The sexual services do not necessarily have to include sexual intercourse or, indeed, payment! . . . Again, working as a sex worker, or in any other capacity, in a brothel is not of itself an offence . . . Owners and managers are definitely liable to the 'exploitation of prostitution' section of the Sexual Offences Act 2003 . . .

In addition, the Sexual Offences Act 1956 section on brothels has been amended following the police successfully lobbying government to increase the 'penalties for keeping a brothel' to cover those cases where they could not prove control. Because the definition of a brothel is so wide – it covers gay saunas, clubs where people have sex on the premises and arguably just about every hotel in the country. The Sexual Offences Act 2003 added a new section 33a to the 1956 Act covering brothels 'to which people resort for practices involving prostitution (whether or not also for other practices)' . . . Maids or housekeepers in brothels are at risk from section 33a, but if your involvement is of a 'menial' nature and you have no control over prices and services, generally you will be committing no offence. It may be useful to have a clear idea of what your duties are to guard against unfair prosecution or conviction.

It is an offence under section 3 of the Children and Young Person Act 1933 to allow a child or young person who is between 4 and 15 inclusive and who you are responsible for to reside in or to frequent a brothel.

Working alone from your own flat, as an independent, is legal with the following provisos. It is legal to provide sexual services in a house or flat as long as there is only one person selling sex. If there are more than that, even *at different times*, the premises can be classified as a brothel and you may be at risk from the Sexual Offences Act 1956 sections 33 and 33a.

Despite the fact that women would be safer if someone else was on the premises, section 33a would charge you with keeping or running a brothel if there were. SW5 says:

Under the Street Offences Act 1959, 'It is an offence for a common prostitute to loiter or solicit in a street or public place for the purpose of prostitution.' A 'common prostitute' has been defined as someone who offers his or her body 'commonly' (ie frequently) for sexual services in return for payment. Men can now be common prostitutes. Loitering or soliciting includes any tempting or alluring of prospective customers, through words, winks, glances, gestures, smiles or provocative movements. You don't have to move: in 1976 someone was found guilty for sitting, stationary, in a window – it was held that she was still tempting clients in for the purpose of prostitution. A 'street or public' place includes any road or lane, subway, court, square, alley, passageway, doorway or entrance to premises adjoining a street. It also covers working from windows and balconies and in public areas of hotels.

Before you can be charged with this, you need to have been given two 'street cautions' within the last year. They are given verbally on location, on the evidence of two or more police officers, and are kept on police records. It is possible to receive both warnings and be charged in a single day or night. If you receive a street caution when you weren't in fact working, you can apply to the Magistrates Court for the area within 14 days to have details of the caution taken off police records. The magistrate will hear evidence from both parties in a private court.

The advantage of this system is that they mean the police must warn you that continued soliciting might lead to an arrest before actually arresting you. The problem is that, as the cautions will be referred to if you are taken to court for soliciting, magistrates may simply 'rubber stamp' police assertions that you were doing so on the occasion in question. It should be up to the police to prove beyond reasonable doubt that you were in fact soliciting on a particular occasion, as opposed to, for example, waiting for a friend. It's worth taking careful note of your circumstances and surroundings at the time of your arrest – for example, the exact whereabouts of this car or that person – to help you to challenge inaccurate assertions. The penalty is a fine.

The unfortunate reality for all women is that you don't actually have to be working the streets to be affected by this legislation, as Carol found out.

In Good Company

A friend of mine, who was a PR person for a reputable company, went to a restaurant that her company wanted to do business with. It was an evening appointment, and she stayed on, had a drink and a chat with them, and then wanted to get home. She just so happened to be blonde, slim, pretty and wearing a nice suit and heels. She called herself a cab and sat on a wall waiting for it to come, and after a while she noticed that the same car kept passing and the men inside it looking at her. About the third time round, they stopped and got out, and she was quite scared – but then they said they were police officers and wanted to know what she was doing and if she was 'working'. She said they were horrible to her, really rude, and she had to go back to the restaurant and get the owner to confirm that she was a PR person waiting for a cab home or they would have arrested her.

If convicted, you can now be placed on the Sex Offenders Register, as SW5 explains:

The Sex Offenders Act 1997, now replaced by the Sexual Offences Act 2003, created what has become known as the Sex Offenders Register. Anyone convicted of any of a number of sexual offences has to register with their local police for a specified number of years. Failure to comply can result in being imprisoned for up to six months. The actual offences vary in Scotland and Northern Ireland, but are broadly similar. In England, Wales and Northern Ireland, accepting a police caution for these offences also carries with it the need to register. *Get legal advice before accepting cautions.* People who have committed sexual crimes abroad (when the act was a crime both in the country concerned and in the UK) or who were found unfit to stand trial or found not guilty through insanity are also liable to be put on the register. If your sentence is 30+ months imprisonment then your time on the Sexual Offenders Register will be for life. If you get 7–29 months it is ten years. 0–6 months is seven years. If you have a conditional discharge then your time on the register is for the period of the conditional discharge. People on the register must notify the police within three days of any move or seven days in advance of any foreign travel for three or more days . . .

New Sexual Offences Prevention Orders replace the earlier Sex Offender Orders. They may be made by a court on conviction for a violent or sexual offence, or following an application by the police in respect of a person with such a conviction living in the community. An order lasts for at least five years and may prohibit the offender from doing anything specified in it thought necessary to protect the public or any particular members of the public from serious sexual harm.

In Good Company

Cari Mitchell from the English Collective of Prostitutes states, 'it is a grave injustice for women convicted of prostitution offences – offences which essentially involve consenting sex – to be classified as sex offenders alongside rapists and other violent men.'[6]

Some more from SW5 on stripping and lap dancing:

> Both are legal. Some lap/table-dancing clubs charge their dancers a fee to work there, and expect them to work for tips alone. Sadly, this is legal – it creates an incentive for the club to have more staff than customer demand would suggest . . .

On telephone sex:

> There are few laws against this. It is illegal under the Post Office Acts to use the public telecommunications network to transmit indecent material.

On porn work:

> provided you are at least 18, it is legal to perform in a porn film or photo shoot . . . the appeals panel of The British Board of Film Classification and the courts agree with juries: unless a film involves children, animals or extreme violence etc, then it should qualify for an R18 certificate. Anyone possessing any indecent images – including entirely fictitious 'pseudo-photographs' – of someone under 18 is com-

mitting a serious offence (unless the person featured is at least 16, married to the person possessing them and they do not involve any third party).

On BDSM work:

If you offer sadomasochistic services involving the infliction of blows or other injuries intended or likely to cause bodily harm which is more than 'transient or trifling', you yourself may be charged with assault. Although assault usually requires an absence of consent, it has been held that it is not in the public interest that a person should harm another in order to gratify sexual desire. Thus the fact that the client requested or consented to the blows, and paid for them, may be no defence.

On drug use:

Sex work can bring you into contact with drugs of all sorts. If these are controlled by the Misuse of Drugs Act 1971, it is a criminal offence to possess them or to share, give or sell them. Drug use in working flats and brothels can attract police attention. If you are working on the streets and the police arrest you for soliciting and you have drugs on you, you may end up being charged with the drugs as well.

In Good Company

On taxation:

> Sex workers are liable to declare their earnings and pay taxes like everyone else. Over the years, several prostitutes have claimed in court that they should not have to pay taxes as that would result in the government 'living on the earnings of prostitution' . . .
>
> The positive side is that as with other businesses you may be entitled to deduct expenses such as the cost of advertising, condoms, lube, toys, magazines, videos, rent etc. Ask around to find a good accountant. If you don't pay income tax and are discovered, the Inland Revenue can present you with a large bill based on their assessment of your undeclared earnings. They can go back a maximum of 12 years, and it's up to you to challenge their figures . . .
>
> If you do come to their attention, voluntarily or otherwise, what the Inland Revenue have tended to do is send an assessment for a ridiculous amount as a way of making sure they don't undercharge you. People in cash industries – like sex work – tend to get particularly silly initial assessments. Why? If you get a bill for tax on £50,000 and you in fact earned £100,000, there is obviously going to be a temptation to say 'yes, that's right' and pay the lower bill. But if it's the other way around, it becomes in your interest (and makes their life easier) to be able to demonstrate that their initial assessment is wrong. And that needs good record keeping – a diary of clients, income, expenditure etc.

Most people's experience is that if you are honest with the Inland Revenue, they are fair in return. If you are not, the Inland Revenue sometimes works in conjunction with the police, accompanying them on raids. It has wide powers of entry of its own.

The Republic of Ireland

Mr McDowell, Minister for Justice, Equality and Law Reform in Ireland, says the following about the laws on prostitution in The Republic of Ireland:

Prostitution is not in itself a crime, but the law seeks to protect prostitutes from exploitation and to protect the public from certain manifestations of prostitution. It is an offence for a person, in a street or public place, to solicit or importune another person for the purposes of prostitution. The offence applies equally to a prostitute soliciting a client, a client soliciting a prostitute or a third party soliciting one on behalf of the other. The same offence and penalties apply to prostitutes, clients or anyone who solicits in a public place. It is also an offence to solicit or importune another person in order to commit certain sexual offences, such as sexual offences with underage persons or to keep or to manage a brothel.

A significant provision is that a member of the Garda Síochána, who has reasonable cause to suspect that a person is loitering in a street or public place in order to solicit for the purpose of prostitution, may direct that person to leave the scene immediately. It is then an offence not to comply with such a direction without reasonable cause. 'Loitering' includes loitering in a motor vehicle and this provision therefore also applies to kerb-crawlers. In addition to its other provisions the Criminal Law (Sexual Offences) Act 1993 also extended the law on soliciting in public, which previously applied only to prostitutes and any third parties organising and profiting from prostitution.[7]

USA

In America:

After 1965, prostitution entered a new period of openness and publicity. One study in 1968 . . . estimated that every day 286,650 men visited prostitutes. Sporadic attempts have been made over the years to legalise prostitution on various grounds, and in 1971 Nevada became the first state to do so (in its smaller counties).

Prostitutes themselves grew more assertive. In 1973, San Francisco's Margo St James, a college-educated prostitute, founded the first labour organisation for prostitutes known as COYOTE (Call Off Your Old Tired Ethics). Similar organisations followed in other states. St James and her supporters defended prostitution as a privacy issue, demanding that it be accepted as legitimate women's work, but feminist and other groups attacked this libertarian view,

charging that prostitution was an exploitative exten-
sion of women's dependency on men. By the end of
the 1980s, however, growing fears regarding the AIDS
epidemic threatened prostitutes with even greater
regulation and discrimination.[8]

According to section 2422 'coercion and enticement' of the
US Penal Code:

(a) Whoever knowingly persuades, induces, entices,
     or coerces any individual to travel in interstate or
     foreign commerce, or in any Territory or
     Possession of the United States, to engage in
     prostitution, or in any sexual activity for which
     any person can be charged with a criminal
     offence, or attempts to do so, shall be fined
     under this title or imprisoned not more than 20
     years, or both.

(b) Whoever, using the mail or any facility or means
     of interstate or foreign commerce, or within the
     special maritime and territorial jurisdiction of the
     United States knowingly persuades, induces,
     entices, or coerces any individual who has not
     attained the age of 18 years, to engage in prosti-
     tution or any sexual activity for which any person
     can be charged with a criminal offence, or
     attempts to do so, shall be fined under this title,
     imprisoned not less than 5 years and not more
     than 30 years.[9]

Article 230 of the New York Penal Code states that: 'A person is guilty of prostitution when such person engages or agrees or offers to engage in sexual conduct with another person in return for a fee. Prostitution is a class B Misdemeanor.'[10] While in California the State code 266 says:

> Every person who inveigles or entices any unmarried female, of previous chaste character, under the age of 18 years, into any house of ill fame, or of assignation, or elsewhere, for the purpose of prostitution, or to have illicit carnal connection with any man; and every person who aids or assists in such inveiglement or enticement; and every person who, by any false pretenses, false representation, or other fraudulent means, procures any female to have illicit carnal connection with any man, is punishable by imprisonment in the state prison, or by imprisonment in a county jail not exceeding one year, or by a fine not exceeding two thousand dollars ($2,000), or by both such fine and imprisonment.[11]

In the US every state sets its own age of consent, which varies from 13 to 18.

New Zealand

In an ideal world every country would be as forward thinking as New Zealand, with its experiment for the last two years in not criminalising women for selling sex, effectively allowing them to legally work for themselves from their own homes. As Catherine Healey of The New Zealand Prostitutes Collective says:

> In New Zealand the key thing about the 2003 Prostitution Reform Act (PRA) is that decriminalisation included decriminalising prostitution on the street. This was a real milestone and our bottom line. Decriminalisation allows for women to work from their own home – some women have come off the street and advertise using their mobile phones. There has been no increase in numbers of women working. Decriminalisation has made a big difference to whether women feel able to report rape and other violence. We have made substantial gains and in some cases have turned police and courts around. Women can now question police actions. Police have to get a warrant to come into premises. Before PRA brothel managers took advantage of women because the work was illegal. We had wide support for this law from MPs, rape crisis organisations, the National Council on Women, Business and Professional Women's Federation, The Maori Women's Welfare League, The Public Health Unit and The NZ AIDS Foundation.[12]

The Prostitution Reform Act of June 2003 repealed the following provisions: section 26 of the Summary Offences Act 1981 (soliciting), section 147 of the Crimes Act 1961 (brothel keeping), section 148 of the Crimes Act 1961 (living on the earnings of prostitution), section 149 of the Crimes Act 1961 (procuring sexual intercourse) and the Massage Parlours Act 1978 and related regulations. The Prostitution Reform Act of 2003 also decriminalises the sale of sex and the ownership and management of a brothel.

It also makes it illegal to cause or assist children to participate in the sex industry. Children are defined as those persons who have not reached 18. The Crimes Act 1961 provides that there is no defence to having sex with an underage person if the person charged believed the child was of age or consented. For consistency, a similar subsection was included in the Prostitution Reform Act.

As humantrafficking.org says:

> The Human Rights Commission supports the Prostitution Reform Act and is of the opinion that the reforms will create an environment that is both less hostile and more transparent to those victimised by the trafficking industry. It prohibits the granting of permits under the Immigration Act based on provision of commercial sex, and prohibits holders of temporary permits from providing commercial sex.[13]

Hopefully what this will mean in practice is that less women will be coerced into the sex industry against their will and that those women who do work within the industry will be able to do so without fear or abuse. It also prohibits anyone who does not have a valid permit to work in the country from gaining a license to provide commercial sex.

The Media and the Law

A Prostitution Law Review Committee will review the operation of the Act within five years, and consider (among other matters) whether any amendments to the law are desirable to limit or control the location and conduct of prostitution.

Australia

In Australia different states have different laws, and in some states prostitution has been totally legalised, meaning that it is no longer an offence to sell sex for money, while in others it has been decriminalised – meaning that while not legal it is not a crime worthy of the law courts and punishment though it generally requires attaining a license from local government.

According to the Maxim Institute:

> prostitution was fully legalised in Victoria in the mid-1980s, ACT in 1992, Queensland in 2000, and decriminalised in NSW in 1995...However, the majority of the sex industry operates in the illegal sector, as licensing and zoning requirements are onerous and expensive. Requirements include mandatory fortnightly health checks for workers, but not for clients. Debbie Neilson, president of the Queensland Adult Business Association, which represents the state's licensed brothel operators, said recently it was impossible to compete with Queensland's massive underground sex industry. She put the ratio of illegal operators to licensed premises at a hundred to one. A *Sydney*

Morning Herald investigation found that the number of establishments operating in Sydney had more than tripled within a few years since decriminalisation.[14]

Raymond Miller, a massage parlour owner for 30 years, quoting for The Maxim Institute, says, 'It can confidently be predicted that decriminalisation will at least double or treble those choosing to operate [as private operators] because the fear of prosecution is removed.'[15]

Tim Barnett a New Zealand MP says:

Prostitution was decriminalised in the Australian state of New South Wales in 1995. There is no system of licensing but brothels are required to comply with the Land and Environment Act and Local Body Authorities Regulations. Home occupation regulations apply to sex work, but there is no registration of sex workers' names (as is the current practice in some places in New Zealand). Street work is generally legal in commercial areas, and operators of venues are required to promote safer sex information and supply safer sex products to workers.[16]

Canada

While prostitution itself is legal in Canada, how it is practised is restricted and enforcement differs greatly in different cities.

Section 213 of the Criminal Code of Canada is the communication law, the aim of which is to avoid street prostitution by preventing soliciting or having sex in public. It states that communicating (in public) for the purpose of prostitution is a summary conviction offence.

As John Lowman of The School of Criminology at Simon Fraser University tells us:

> In addition to the communicating law, 'bawdy houses' are prohibited (Criminal Code sections 210 and 211), as are procuring and living on the avails of prostitution of another person (section 212). Procuring and living on the avails are indictable offences carrying terms of up to ten years in prison (and in the case of a person under 18, up to 14 years in prison). A common bawdy house is a place kept, occupied or used by at least one person for the purposes of prostitution or indecent acts. 'Keeping' a bawdy house (section 210(1)) is an indictable offence liable to up to two years in prison. Being 'found in' or an 'inmate' of a bawdy house (Criminal Code sections 210(2) and 211) are summary offences carrying a maximum term of six months in prison and/or a $2,000 fine (being a summary offence, the communicating law carries the same maximum penalties).

The living on the avails, procuring and bawdy house laws date back to Canada's first criminal code, as did the vagrancy provision which prohibited street prostitution. The vagrancy law was replaced in 1972 with the soliciting law which, in turn, was replaced by the communicating law.[17]

In Good Company

According to the Canadian Sex Work Cyber Resource And Support Center:

Under the Canadian Criminal Code:

(1) The act of prostitution is legal, ie you cannot be arrested for being a prostitute.

(2) The practice of independent outcall prostitution is fully protected by Federal law. Third party involvement in solicitation of business or profiting from it is a crime but enforcement varies widely since the attitude is to support individual rights as long as it doesn't hurt anyone else.

(3) Advertising in public print is protected as a right of free speech which has been upheld by the Canadian Supreme Court. Advertising on television has not yet been tested but the issue is whether it's in line with community standards.

(4) An independent outcall escort has the right to discuss specific acts of sex for money in private. Hotel rooms, telephones and private homes. The Canadian Supreme court has ruled that a land based telephone is a private communication. When one places a phone call, they have a reasonable expectation of privacy, and that is the test. The same is easily extended to cellular phone communication. One would have to have special equipment to intercept such communication.

When you consider the 'public communication' aspect of the law it is really crafted to discourage street solicitation. The more aggressive uses of the law have seen it applied to hotel bars, your vehicle, operating on a public street and other such places. Communication by the way also includes acts in furtherance as evidence of intent . . . ie you pick a street walker up in your car is an act of furtherance.[18]

France

Despite France's long history of legal prostitution, in 2003 they passed The Internal Security Act which, amongst other things, recriminalised prostitution. Many sex workers, according to the Green Left organisation, believe that this was done primarily as a way of coping with France's immigration problems, though Nicholas Sarkozy, the man who pushed this Act through the French National Assembly, claimed in 2004 that it had reduced prostitution by 40 per cent:

French law defines soliciting as publicly inciting another person by any means, including by clothing or attitude, to have sexual intercourse, in exchange for financial remuneration or a promise of such remuneration.[19]

According to Alex Lefebvre on the World Socialist website:

The law targets prostitution, making it a crime punishable by two months in jail and a 3,750-euro fine to publicly invite someone to have sexual relations even passively, by one's attitude.[20]

In Good Company

Many governments' attitudes towards prostitution can be compared to that of the local council-employed leaf blower – someone paid to push the obvious problem under a bush or carpet, moving the 'problem' out of sight so that it would seem that it does not exist. This is palpably an attitude without logic, sense or foresight. We do not want to be ghettoised. Legalisation and the economic viability to enable women to do what they want with their bodies and their lives are needed throughout the world now. The only way to stop women becoming victims in a society that sees them as second-class citizens is to give them the tools and the rights to shape their own lives.

Chapter Seven

A Guide for Clients

I wrote this book for women but I am expecting that some men will pick it up and glance through it. It's about sex, of course they will. If you are, or wish to become a client, or you are just curious about sex or women in the sex industry, then this chapter is for you.

How you treat women in general is how you should treat any sex worker. People, all people, respond to courtesy and respect. Good manners are not difficult to learn and if applied to everything one does can have a truly beneficial effect on the way others interact with you. Booking and seeing an escort really is not very much different to booking your car into a mechanics or booking a restaurant. If you ring a mechanic and you are a pain in the arse on the phone, chances are your car will take longer to fix and the charge will be higher 'for extra labour, mate'. If you book a table at a restaurant and give the receptionist a hard time for whatever reason, it is possible that you will be seated by the men's toilet and wait ages to be served. The same thing applies to escorts – if you speak with an agency and/or an escort be polite, charming even, and you will generally get a far better time for your money, be treated with respect and get what you want.

Many men could do a lot worse than read Marc Perkel's interesting and informative website about the correct way to deal with sex and sex workers, http://sex.perkel.com/escort/index.htm, written by a man, for men. Marc has reputedly been using the services of escorts and prostitutes for most of his adult life, so if you don't believe what I have to say in this chapter about the way to treat women, in and out of the industry, then take it from him.

Seeing and paying for an escort in the UK is not illegal – you are purchasing time; though it is illegal for women to solicit and for men to 'kerb-crawl' or to pimp women. And, as we saw in Chapter Three with Henry's story (page 86), 'kerb-crawling' can get you into trouble if you approach the wrong individual. I really do not recommend hiring some-one straight off the street.

How To Pick The Right Escort For You

There are many ways to access escorts. You can look for them in the *Yellow Pages*. You can find their advertisements in the back of tourist guides, local newspapers and top shelf magazines. In London you can even walk into a phone box or past a newsagent's window and see a multitude of cards offering an array of 'services' (not recommended in my opinion). If you don't care who you see then the above options are fine; telephone the agency in question and ask for someone. But the best way is through the internet. This way you can actually see what is on offer. Go to any search engine and type in 'escort agency' and the city you are in. They will give you an overwhelming response. At the time of writing, typing 'escort agency + London' into Google gets you a staggering 1,390,000 results, try 'escort agency + New York' and you get 839,000, while 'escort agency + Sydney' gets you 214,000.

Don't be overwhelmed, click on any link you like and it will take you somewhere that, if not what you are looking for, will inevitably lead you somewhere else through their large 'links page'.

Most escort agencies will have an introduction page, generally with a standard disclaimer about the fact that they are only providing time and companionship and that if anything else occurs it is between the escort and the individual; a gallery page, where you can see thumbnail images of the women on their books; click on the thumbnails and you will find a page for each escort, which will have a few more images, quite often bigger than thumbnail size, a general description of her and what services she offers and her rates; and a links page, which as previously stated will take you to any number of other related sites. Shop around a bit on the internet unless you see your 'ideal' woman immediately.

Be aware that not all of what you see is ethical or true. Some adult sites are 'mirror' sites, that is they have several URLs that all go to the one agency. Some sites are merely fronts for pay per view porn so never give your credit card details to an adult site unless you know exactly what you are getting and feel comfortable with their security arrangements. (In June 2003 in the UK the losses to credit card fraud were £128.8 million – 3 per cent of this was attributed to the internet. In the US the amount of online fraud in 2004 came to US$1,456.92million.[1]) Some sites use images of women that are not real. Some adult sites are even 'homes' for virus – I recommend the use of a 'pop up stopper' when accessing adult sites that you are not familiar with.

The only real way to find out if what you are seeing online is what you can actually get is by contacting them by telephone or email. If you telephone be aware of how the phone is answered. If a well-spoken voice answers with 'Good evening, Escort Agency, how can I help' you are probably onto a reputable agency. Do not be afraid to ask questions, but bear in mind that the person on the other end of the phone line does not know who you are and may be a little cagey (see the information on entrapment in Chapter Six). (There will be more on what to say and how to say it in the next section.) Most, but not all, escort agencies do not have a huge group of women sitting around and waiting for your all-important call. A good agency will take your details – if you want someone to visit you they will want your name, address and landline or hotel room number. If they don't ask for this and they do not explain that they will run a check to see you are who you say you are then you may be dealing with an agency that does not give a damn about its girls and is therefore somewhat suspect. They will then contact the escort of your choice and either send her straight to you or get her to telephone you. If you do not hear back from the agency or the escort within 10–15 minutes then you are probably dealing with time-wasters.

Sadly, many agencies all over the world work from a stance of deliberate exploitation. Many charge their workers excessive amounts of commission; some will take a cheque upfront from you the client and then just not pay the girl at all. The best way to judge whether these things are likely to be happening is the way in which you are asked to pay for your experience. It should always be directly to the escort, in cash and immediately before your time with her begins. Any other form of requested payment should set your alarm bells ringing.

You get what you pay for. If you want to spend time with a self-assured sexy intelligent woman of the world then her fee per hour will reflect that. On the other hand, if you want to spend time with a potentially screwed-up female who may be being forced into seeing you by an unscrupulous agent then the chances are she will be an awful lot cheaper. If an escort works for an agency, as opposed to independently, know that she will be paying some percentage of what you give her to that agency, so if you are paying £100 or US$50 per hour you are more likely to get the latter kind of escort than if you were paying £250 or US$400 plus per hour. The choice is yours but the rise of the independent escort has been primarily due to ethical escort clients becoming appalled by the greed and exploitation of agencies over the last five years. This has shown itself in most agencies' accounts books, particularly in London.

How to Communicate with an Escort Agency

We sex workers are not ogres. We want to provide you with what you want and we want to be paid adequately for what we do, and we will be sensitive and understanding of almost anything you have to say, provided you say it politely.

So, you have seen someone you like on the internet and you have phoned the agency or woman in question. Please do not withhold your number. Be polite and circumspect – something like, 'Would it be possible to make an appointment with Danielle this evening?' is just fine. A good agent will tell you straight away if the person you want is available or not. They will then find out if you would like an incall, which means you go to visit the escort at her premises, or an outcall, where she comes to your home or hotel room. If you require a residential outcall then the agency will want your full real name, your address, your landline number, who the landline is registered to and whether it is an ex-directory number. This information will then be checked out by the agency by ringing directory enquires. Should you require a hotel outcall you will be asked for your full name and your hotel room number. The same procedure applies. If you book an incall you will be given an idea of the area of the city where your escort's 'apartment' is and asked to be

A Guide for Clients

in the area ten minutes before your appointed booking time. At that time you phone the agency and they will give you the address.

Please do not discuss straight away with the agent what you want sexually – this is legally and essentially between you and the escort – but if you feel a rapport with the person on the phone and your requirements are somewhat unusual then you can save everyone a lot of time by explaining to the agent that you like 'Greek' or a girl with 'A-Levels' or that you want to be dominated. A good agent will know her escorts and will then be able to say to you that while, yes, the girl you like the look of is available she does not provide the service you want. A good agent will then try to recommend someone to you who might not only fall in with your physical and aesthetic requirements but who will also give you the services you require. This saves time for all concerned, including you, but really should be done with discretion. If your chosen escort is available and telephones you to discuss in more detail what you would like from and with her please feel free to be honest but do it with charm. This is also the time to let the escort know if you have any other requirements like clothing, toys or scenarios. If your experience just won't be the same unless the woman is wearing black stockings and a suspender belt ask the escort on the phone to either wear or bring those items. Should you need to change the time of your appointment or have been asked to confirm your booking you do so through the agent.

The more notice you give an agency and an escort the more likely you are to get exactly what you want. Many

escorts do other things. Some are students, some are
mothers, some have careers, and all have lives. If you want
a specific individual or service, the more notice you give the
more likely you are to get what you want.

How To Prepare Yourself For Your Date

Whenever you find yourself in the company of women,
whether it is an escort you have booked or a girl you have
met in a bar and made a date with, always make a bit of an
effort with your personal appearance and hygiene. If you
have booked for an escort to visit you make sure that both
you and the environment are conducive to having a good
time. Make sure the bed is made and has clean sheets; if it
is evening, light a few candles – particularly if you are not
especially comfortable with your own appearance; buy a
bottle of wine and a bottle of mineral water. Although all
good escorts should carry condoms, place a couple by the
bed just in case, that way if she arrives without them it will
not eat into any of your precious time with her by one of you
having to go out and get them. Shower 15 minutes before
your escort/date arrives. Brush your teeth and your hair.
Have the escort's fee ready and waiting for her when she
arrives. Fritz, a serial escort client, tells us how he operates:

> I have an escort come to my apartment about
> once a fortnight. I always dim the lights, have a
> nice bottle of red wine open for her, sometimes I
> will make a little pasta or salad so she can sit and

relax while we get to know each other. I always shower just before the appointed arrival time and I always offer the girl the opportunity to do so when she arrives. Sometimes, even if I have had my shower, I shower again with the escort – that can be fun.

If you have booked an incall and you are, for example, coming straight from work, and consequently cannot get cleaned up before you arrive at her place, ask her on arrival, after you have paid her the fee, if you could possibly use her shower. She will be impressed at your politeness and pleased that you want to make the effort. She might even give you a bit of a scrub down! As Celia explains:

I always make them shower and I keep a stock of about 20 toothbrushes; I put a new one out for every client that visits me. I love kissing but there is nothing worse than kissing someone who reeks, let alone having sex with them!

How To Treat an Escort

If your escort provides a GFE (Girl Friend Experience) then she will be quite happy to kiss and cuddle on meeting you. Get the cash transacting out of the way straight away, then she will have to ring her agency to let them know that she has arrived, that you are okay and that she has the money. This is where the fun starts. If you have already discussed your requirements on the phone then it can be quite easy to go straight into whatever roles you both want to play. If you haven't then sit back, get comfortable and relate to her what ever you want. This will get you both feeling horny and should find you getting into the 'swing of things' within minutes. If all you want to do is sit and chat for the time that she is there, that is all right too.

Never force an escort to do anything she does not want to do. Remember that most escorts, through virtue of their profession, are quite likely to be far more sexually experienced than you and many have a lot of 'tricks' up their sleeves for making a man feel sexy and good – see what an escort can teach you if you don't have any specific requirements in mind. Treat her with respect and your experience will be improved tenfold.

Booking an escort is like booking and paying for any other service. The fact that companionship and, more often than not, sex is the commodity does not lessen the person providing the service. Consistently treat all women well and with respect, and I promise you will reap the benefits.

Afterthoughts – Were You Happy?

After the 'date' is over men seem to experience a variety of different feelings. Most seem to go to sleep but some experience an overwhelming sense of guilt. Some feel huge elation, others feel angry. If you are one of those men that experiences guilt then please let go of it. You have done nothing more or less than carry out a commercial transaction that has benefited you enormously – like going to a physiotherapist or an osteopath when you have put your back out. You have paid for someone effectively to soothe your ache or fill your loneliness and you have done so honestly. You haven't coerced anyone into bed with you. You haven't gone out or gone home and raped anyone. You have not committed the most heinous crime of the century. You have merely paid for an escort.

However, if you find yourself becoming slightly addicted to escorts but you cannot lose the guilt then it might be time for you to reconsider your options and lifestyle, as Christian did:

> I live in a small town with my family. Every week for about six months I felt compelled to go to London and hire an escort. I had to hide the money from my family. I had to lie about where I was and what I was doing. I got so obsessed I nearly lost my business. Sometimes I would see the same girl week after week, sometimes it would be a different one every week. Eastern European blondes generally. Eventually I realised something was really up with me. I called the agency I used after one particular booking and confessed my torturous feelings of guilt. The woman there was lovely and very understanding. She told me that I had not done anything wrong but that if I was continually feeling this bad about it then maybe I should consider taking a break for a while to see how I felt. I took her advice

and I have not seen an escort for four months. I
miss the experience but my business and family life
are back on track and I do not feel like I am going
crazy anymore.

Whether your experience was a happy one or not you
should first of all telephone the agency. Escort agencies
and escorts love genuine feedback. An agency needs to
know if, on the one hand, an escort has stolen something
from you or tried to over charge you for 'extras' not previously discussed, or, on the other hand, if your experience
was so mindblowingly wonderful that it 'was the best sex
you ever had'. An agency that knows these things can act
on them effectively. If an escort gets a glowing review from
a client she and her agency can use that on her web page.
If she has done something negative then the agency can
either discuss this with her or potentially not get her any
more work. Agencies want your feedback so don't hesitate
to give it to them.

The other thing you can do is post a review on a website
purpose-built for just this. There are quite a few but the
main ones are www.captain69.co.uk and www.punter
net.com. Or in America there is RAPS (The Review and
Posting Society) at www.aspd.net.

Captain 69 is a well-established site that covers the
whole world and almost every aspect of the escorting industry. It boasts a comprehensive database of escorts and
agencies, listing not only by country but also by body, hair
and service type. You do have to pay to join and membership

entitles you, amongst other things, to write and read reviews. The site is thoroughly comprehensive and I recommend anyone interested in escorts and escorting to use it.

Punternet first went online in 1999. According to it's Webmaster and 'personality', Galahad, the 'site was created to facilitate the exchange of information on prostitution in the UK' and provides 'information on where to find services, what to expect, legalities, etc. You will be able to read reviews of encounters with working girls and submit your own "field reports".' It is free to read what Galahad calls 'field reports' and there is a simple and free registration in order to be able to post up your own field report. He is also happy to post escort 'rebuttals' to field reports. Like Captain 69, they have a comprehensively huge database, but do seem to be more focused on the UK.

RAPS is a comprehensive American site that enables the user to get reviews by city and state. It also has an international section. Viewing and reading most of the site is free as is registering so that one can contribute oneself, although more membership 'privileges' can be attained by paying.

Before you write a review remember that you can, in effect, make or break an escort's career. Post a bad review and hundreds, if not thousands of people will read it with the consequence that that escort may not ever get work under that persona again (see Katrina's story in Chapter Two – page 61). If you have had a genuinely bad experience and you feel that the agency involved did not take you seriously, by all means tell the truth in the forums provided, but please don't post a bad review out of malice or because an escort won't see you again. Becoming an escort is more often than not a financial consideration – please think very carefully before you damage someone's economic viability. On the other hand if you have had an amazing time, please do tell people about it in the appropriate forum – you will help that particular escort on to a whole new working plateau. Most escorts who get a lot of work do so because their reputations precede them. A good reputation in this industry is worth its weight in gold both to escorts and clients alike.

What Clients Should Not Do

While many men using the services of escorts are polite and courteous, many more are not. Both agencies and independents receive far more communication from people who are not serious and who are not as pleasant as they could be, so here are a few guidelines of what not to do:

Do not ring an agency when you are inebriated. Any responsible agent will not take your details if they suspect you of being too drunk or coked off your face to either maintain politeness or get it up. I, personally as an agent, would not contact a girl for you if you were rude, discourteous, plainly drunk or offensive to me. I mean, why would I bother? I would, conversely, be incredibly polite to you but I would not make any effort to assuage your needs or desires. Instead, when I had got off the phone I would put you in my little black book of clients who are: rude, offensive, violent, abusive, rip off girls, refuse to wear condoms, try using counterfeit money, book but don't show etc. I would then contact my rather extensive network of other sex workers and relay that information to them. The consequence of which, if I need to spell it out, is that should you genuinely wish to book an escort it may prove rather difficult. I hear men muttering 'So? There are hundreds of escorts in every city and town in the world' and they are right, but bear in mind – you get what you pay for. Sex workers do network with each other; we do pass information to each other all the time. If you live in one city and you don't travel a lot and you wish to use the services of escorts at a particular financial level don't piss them off because the word will get around.

Do not give false personal information. Desiring a woman to visit you does mean that you do have to give your address, and the agency will check out your details so you will need to give your real name. Simple and obvious though this seems, many men have problems coping with this small fundamental. Only this morning at 3 am a 'gentleman' called my own agency requiring someone to visit him. The procedure was explained and he stated that he understood. However the conversation went something like this: 'Can I take your name?' 'Urghhaaahh.' 'I'm sorry could you repeat that?' 'Hmm, Benjamin.' 'Is that your first or second name?' 'What?' 'Could I take your second name?' 'Harry' 'Okay, Benjamin, can I take your address?' 'That's a bit personal isn't it?'. All you will have done by providing false information is wasted your phone call and the agent's time, which will not endear you to them should you wish to genuinely book an escort through them again.

Do not call on a withheld number. This may seem very simplistic to you but appears to be shockingly necessary to point out. I know of several independent escorts who now no longer keep their mobile phones switched on because of the amount of time-wasting calls that they receive. They will check their voicemails every half hour to see if any genuine clients have called. It is not just independent escorts, many agencies too will not answer calls from withheld numbers. The implication being that if you cannot give your phone number then you cannot be considered a safe client. Also, due to the sad nature of our society, it would seem that many men are what I call left handed mouse users. You know who you are. You are alone and you are masturbating over the images you see on the internet. If you have no intention of booking an escort, if all you really want is to wank while a woman speaks to you on the telephone then please do us all a favour and give a dedicated phone sex line a call. In the same vein be aware that most agencies have one person answering all the individual escorts emails. If you are genuine do not email ten different girls all at the same agency, all with the same email. They will assume you are another time-waster!

Don't call until you are ready. The other big no-no is what I call the silent fear – if you are too nervous to speak to an agent or an escort please do not dial their number until you are feeling more confident. On average I receive five to ten calls a day from people unable to open their mouths and verbalise, they either hang up straight away or breathe pathetically. If you are genuinely nervous, if this is your first time, be honest. We won't bite. Not unless you want us to.

Do not be explicit or crude. Please do not ask an agency if the girl of your choice 'will take it up the arse'! When speaking with an escort bear in mind that saying, 'I was wondering if you would consider A', is far more likely to get you what you want than: 'So, can I stick it up your back passage'.

Do not expect and do not ask for an escort's phone number.

Do not expect instant availability if you are not prepared to be flexible about your requirements. If you want someone at your hotel in half an hour prepare to not be fussy about whom you see. There is absolutely no point in whining at an agency because you want to see Jessica in half an hour at 5 pm in central London when the agency has already told you that Jessica is a student and will not be available until after 7.30 pm. She may be able to make it at 5 pm if you give her 24 hours notice; or listen to the agent's recommendation of who can be there in the timescale you have given.

Do not expect two for the price of one. If you want to see two escorts at the same time whether it be for a 'bisexual show' or because you feel you have a sexual libido that needs two women for you to be satisfied, then know that this will double your costs. Two escorts equals two fees. Please do not demean the escorts, the agency or yourself by expecting a discount.

Do not arrive unwashed. Smelly, sweaty men with bad breath do not turn any woman on. Please be clean.

In Good Company

Do not expect extra time for free. If you have booked and paid for an hour do not try to coerce the escort to stay with you for longer unless you have the requisite cash to buy or pay for more of her time. If she is with a reputable agency they will be expecting her to ring them on the hour. If you disable her from doing so the agency will try to contact you. If they cannot get hold of either you or their escort after a pre-arranged amount of time then they may well call the police. It is not in anyone's interest for you not to allow the escort to ring the agency on the hour or for you to try to get her so drunk that she forgets to do so.

Do not ask a sex worker for unsafe sex. She will turn you down.

Do not make a booking if you do not intend to keep it. If you are unable to keep a genuine appointment please have the courtesy to notify either the escort or the agency.

Chapter Eight

Making The Most of Being an Escort

Hopefully you will have read this book and realised whether sex industry work is right for you. If it is, the primary things to know are: don't allow yourself to be coerced into anything you do not want to do, do your research well, listen to your instincts and maintain your self-respect at all times. If the horror stories contained in this book, all of which are true stories, have made you realise that the work is not for you that is all well and good, but as you go through your everyday life working in any 'profession' I believe the same principles should apply. Never allow yourself to be bullied or become the 'victim' of workplace harassment; if you really want something then go for it; believe in yourself and your right to be able to live and work without poverty or fear. Help other women to achieve the same things.

If, having read through this book, you find that you would like to give escorting a go, even if it is just once to assuage some sexual fantasy that you may have been harbouring for years, then follow the advice given earlier carefully.

In Good Company

Always listen to your 'inner voice'. Listen to it and you might have fun and make a bit of money, as Alina did. Though I personally don't condone her method, there is no denying she got what she wanted:

I was 19 years old and it was my second night of working in a brothel ever. Two wealthy Arab brothers walked in wanting a girl to stay with them in a hotel above Jupiter's Casino on the Gold Coast in Surfer's Paradise for eight days. They selected me and made me an offer. We would all be having our own rooms. I would get $5,000 for a wardrobe of clothes and $15,000 to stay in the hotel and have sex with them. They also offered me an extra $15,000 to have sex without a condom. I agreed. I know this was crazy but the money was blinding me. We drove off in a limo. They were both similar looking, they both had eight-inch cocks and they both performed the same in bed. My days panned out like this – I would get up in the morning and put my hair up and dress in a classy suit with high heels. I would go downstairs and join them in the limo. The day was spent having meetings and looking at property as they were in Australia to buy property. We would return to the hotel in the late afternoon. I would have a drink and a meal on my own and return to my room where I would freshen up, put on sexy clothes and boots, let my long blonde hair down and wait for their call. At about

Making The Most of Being an Escort

8 pm one of the brothers would call. I would go to his room, disrobe slowly and have sex with him. During the course of the evening he would come at least a couple of times, then I would return to my room at about 11 pm. Exactly the same thing happened every day and every night, with the brothers alternating the evenings. This went on for eight days from one brother to the other. $35,000 for a week's work. Better than being on the dole!

Never have unsafe sex.

Ignore your inner voice and you may find yourself becoming yet another tragic casualty of an industry that has no shortage of martyrs. Tamara cannot tell her own story because she currently resides in a 'mental health unit', which she cannot leave and to which people from her past are not allowed to visit, but I knew her well:

Tamara grew up in a Pakistani family in London's East End. Neither of her parents spoke English. From the age of five she was sexually abused by uncles and then by older brothers. As a young and quite wild teenager she was torn between her family's culture and her peers on the streets outside. At the age of 14 three men in a London park raped her. When she informed her family, she was vilified (because she must have encouraged it) and thrown out of their home. She started doing glamour modelling at the age of 15 after being picked up while out shopping by an 'agent', this in turn led on to two porn films. I met Tamara when she was 19 and applied for a job with the agency I was then managing. She was an escort agent's dream – tiny but perfectly formed, beautiful, exotic and vivacious. She got a lot of work, seeing a client almost every day. She got great reviews on Captain 69. After about six months it became obvious to me that she was doing far too many drugs. She had always smoked weed but was now also doing large amounts of cocaine. She became more and more erratic. Forgetting to call in from jobs, forgetting she had a job when she had spoken to the client only half an hour before, forgetting to bank her commissions. It all came to a head one sunny Saturday afternoon. Tamara was found naked on her doorstep, screaming: 'I could solve all the world's problems by fucking all the men of power.' This was a litany she would repeat over and over again for months. Her family were called and one of her older sisters had her committed. She was sectioned for three months but during that time, on numerous occasions, she attempted to run away, hurt other people in the unit and accused everyone around her of stealing and 'not knowing who she was'.

Tamara's story cannot be fully blamed on her time in the sex industry but I believe it did not help when deposited on a foundation of sexual abuse (both within the family environment and out of it), cultural uncertainty and teenage angst.

If you are in the industry already and working for an unscrupulous person or agency I hope that you find yourself able to make the break – if more women valued themselves more highly then those who would exploit and abuse us would have less opportunity to do so. People of this nature could not get away with it if we did not allow them to. By giving someone 50 per cent of your earnings, by doing things you do not want to do without standing up and saying no, by devaluing yourself below a self-respecting rate, you are effectively confirming to all of the greedy, loathsome people who prey on the vulnerable that it is okay for them to do so. It is not. If you are working for an agency that you feel is ripping you off, leave them. If you are asked either by a client or an agent to do something you don't want to do, politely decline and walk away. Report any instance of sexual or physical abuse to the police. If you are in a situation that you feel you are unable to get out of, for whatever reason, seek help – there are many resources in the back of this book but most cities the world over have women's advice centres and refuges. There are counselling services in most places for women with dependency problems, whether that dependency is drugs, alcohol or sex-related. You are not alone but you do have to speak out to be heard. Do not allow yourself to be made a victim. Stand up and shout and other women will help you. If you are in the unfortunate position of being in a country where you are not legally resident, and are being exploited because of this fact, please seriously analyse what would be a worst-case scenario for you. If the life you are leading currently is bearable then fine, but if it is not would a return to your own country and family, whatever the economic or political situation, be preferable to staying and enduring some form of sexual slavery? Only you can decide this but if your current life is not happy or secure, please get help. Contact the police or your embassy. Contact a women's refuge. Do not allow yourself to be any person's slave. Every individual has the right to freedom.

Over the last five years, the nature of the escort industry, particularly in London, has changed. Because of the unscrupulous nature of many escort agencies the 'client culture' has adapted and absorbed this. Many clients simply do not trust that a girl with an agency will get to keep the money he gives her and that she is actually there with him of her own free will. To any intelligent man paying for 'companionship' this can be the ultimate turn-off. Most escort clients do not want a downtrodden victim of another man's greed, they want a sexy self-assured 'model' who they can interact and have fun with. Because of this the rise of the independent escort has come about.

If you are serious about making money, a lot of money, then the only way to do it is to go independent. This is a step not to be taken lightly. It takes a supreme amount of confidence, a lot of will power and brains. Titania, an independent escort who earns on average a £1,000 per day, says:

Making The Most of Being an Escort

> I lead a good life but I am not extravagant. I have a good car, a lovely home in the country, I work out of a luxury centrally located apartment and I go abroad on holiday every other month. But I do not throw my money around, all the things I have are integral to my work. I know that when I am ready to stop working I will have enough money to retire to the Mediterranean.

Save some of your money. Try to put aside about 50 per cent of what you actually earn. When the commodity is youth and beauty be under no illusions about the fact that it will run out and entering the 'everyday' workplace in your mid-thirties with no other experience than in the sex industry can be quite daunting. Which is not to say that you cannot consider escorting after you turn 30 – many older 'courtesans' do well because their clients remain with them.

I would not advise any woman to go straight into the sex industry on her own. Find an agency run with ethics and learn your business and your craft well. Know the laws of the country or state that you work in and be prepared for the consequences of potentially breaking those laws. Talk with other sex workers to find out which employers and clients are all right and which are not.

Sex workers talk with each other, we have a profoundly far-reaching network – because we are often marginalised by the 'normal' world we have found that communication between ourselves is an effective of way of coping with some of the more negative things that occur in our profession. In my own city if any sex worker I know encounters a 'bad' client then his name, phone number and 'misdemeanour' will be spread across the city's sex workers within an hour. Many independent escorts visiting clients in foreign countries will contact another independent living and working in that country to find out if the client has any kind of reputation.

In fact, it is this communication and sense of mutual responsibility, almost a solidarity, which has kept me working in the industry for as long as I have. For the most part we keep silent about what we do in the hope that the world will not 'out' us and will let us get on with living our lives, but in writing this book I have come to realise that if more women supported each other and helped each other out, communicated with each other and shared their life experiences, we would all be much stronger, individually and collectively. No one ever said life would be easy and for most of us it isn't. There is never enough money to either live well or even, for many women, to rise above the poverty trap. There are endless drudge jobs without intellectual or personal fulfilment. But the more control we take for ourselves, the more we can live without being dependent on anyone else for our survival, the happier we will be as individuals and as women.

Everything in this life should ultimately be your own choice. We know that we do not have a choice about whether we should pay our bills or not but you do have a choice about how you find the money to pay those bills. If we have children we have no other choice but to look after and care for them but you can make choices that will affect their day-to-day existence. Make your choices wisely and from an informed position. Always seek to know more about everything. We live in a time where the dissemination of information freely has never been greater – take advantage of it.

Respect yourself and others. Respect is a viral thing – the more people come into contact with it the more it rubs off. You cannot expect to be respected if you do not have any respect for yourself and you cannot expect others to show you respect if you cannot find it in you to show it to them. Be proud of who you are, whatever you do; be the best that you can be with everyone that you come into contact with and with everything that you do, and do it honestly. In my own experience, life is full of people who will try to convince you that you are not worthy of respect, they will do this in many ways – from the physically or intellectually violent partner who demeans your confidence daily, to the work colleague who tells you that you are not clever enough to get a promotion, to the parent who convinces you that you will not cope in the 'outside world' if you leave home at the age of 26 – but if you believe in yourself strongly enough, these people will drift out of your life before you even realise they are gone because you will have moved on and they will be standing staring at the place you once occupied, wondering where you are.

Be aware of all the things that can go wrong and do your utmost to safeguard against them. How many times have we all said to ourselves 'I know I should have done this, or not done that, but I just didn't think at the time'? As we saw with Becky's story in Chapter Two (page 57), she knew that there had been warning signs and she ignored them. This does not excuse the behaviour of the client in question, which was appalling, but it does serve to show us that not setting yourself up for trouble when your instincts and brain know that something is not quite right is obviously sensible.

All the pieces of advice in this book have been tried and tested. We have the self-imposed rules that we have because they keep us safe. We don't see clients whose information we cannot check or confirm because that is how prostitute women end up dead or raped. We do not give out our phone numbers because sad lonely men will hound or stalk us. We do not give too much of what we do away to others because we do not wish to be judged. We do not give too much of our real selves away to clients because we want to keep our interactions and transactions with them purely commercial. Almost all rules are made to be somewhat bendable – but before you bend any of the rules laid out in this book too hard remember that you only have one life and that you are primarily responsible for it.

If you have read this book and it sits well enough in your psyche that you want to enter the sex industry on any level I say to you: good luck, have fun, make money and, above all, take care. If you have read it and conversely your entire being is screaming, 'Oh no! I couldn't possibly do that!' then don't worry – the sex industry is simply not for you. It really isn't for everyone but please spare a positive thought for all women working and surviving everywhere, no matter how they do it.

The Checklist

For Yourself

- Know the legal reality in your own country
- Keep your alcohol and drug intake to a minimum, particularly when you are on call or with a client
- Maintain your self-respect at all times
- Don't do anything you don't want to do
- Don't do anything just because someone tells you to
- Listen to your own instincts always
- Never undervalue yourself
- Be organised and logical
- If you go independent always check your client's details
- Always practise safe sex
- Always use a condom
- Think very carefully before you tell people what you do
- If you are a student don't escort during exam time
- Own a mobile phone and never switch it off
- Do not take any form of abuse

In Good Company

- Always carry with you: condoms, lubricant, make-up, stockings and suspenders, a change of knickers, sea sponges, a street map of your city, enough cash for a taxi, your mobile phone charger, and, most importantly, paper and pen to write the details of jobs down with
- Have regular STI checks
- Always carry a spray bottle or can of strong, preferably cheap and nasty-smelling perfume, hairspray or some other substance
- Learn self-defence in at least one of its many forms
- Get lots of sleep
- Save some of your money

Dealing with Agencies
- Initially, be discreet
- Always ring in and out of jobs at the required time
- Be wary of male-run agencies
- Do not pay a registration fee
- Be punctual
- Be honest about your personal parameters
- Do not play the 'casting couch' game
- Communicate constantly, particularly when you have a booking
- Always tell your agency about any 'bad' client
- Always tell your agency if you think a client is becoming obsessed in any way with you
- Do not accept 'post payment' by cheque
- Pay your commission as agreed with your agency

The Checklist

Dealing with Clients
- Be a good actress
- Never accept a booking that your agency or yourself have not checked out adequately
- Always withhold your phone number
- Only accept cash upfront – anything else is a freebie
- Check your cash when you get it to ensure that it is kosher
- Keep your money with you at all times
- Only ever take your fee from one person alone
- Only except your local currency unless you or your agency are in a position to do a currency convert
- For incalls never give the client the address until he is five to ten minutes away from the booking
- On hotel bookings always be aware of where the client's room is situated before you get there
- Never go through a hotel reception looking 'tarty' – carry a briefcase and look 'smart/casual'
- Be tolerant and understanding
- Never do anything you do not want to do
- Be discreet
- Be honest about what you will and will not do
- Again, always practise safe sex – always use a condom
- Do not purchase drugs for clients
- Do not consume anything that will cloud your judgement when you are with a client
- Never allow yourself to be locked in a room where you cannot get out of your own volition
- Always know your exits and always have a 'change of plan' strategy

In Good Company

- Always have the wherewithal to get yourself home
- Do not give too much of your personal life away
- Do not overcharge

Resources

Prostitution
UK
The English Collective of Prostitutes
The Crossroads Women's Centre, 230a Kentish Town
Road NW5 2AB
t: 020 7482 2496, minicom: 020 7482 2496
f: 020 7209 4761
ecp@allwomencount.net
Phone lines open: Mon–Fri, 10 am – 4 pm
Open for callers: Tues–Wed 12 – 4 pm
Contact: Niki Adams, Sara Walker, Cari Mitchell
Postal address: Crossroads Women's Centre, PO Box 287,
NW6 5QU
A women's centre where you can get help and advice on all
issues to do with women and children's rights, sex work and
social and financial issues.

In Good Company

Escort Watch

www.escortwatch.co.uk.

A great website where women who work in the industry can communicate with each other and post messages and warnings. In their own words: 'EscortWatch UK is a wholly independent website run for the benefit of those involved in the provision and use of escorting services in the UK and the related industry that has grown up round them . . . We will continue to report on incidents such as violence towards "sex-workers" and electronic abuse so easily suffered from those who use the anonymity of the internet to intimidate and upset. We also wish to be balanced so will also have no hesitation on reporting on cases where clients have suffered at the hands of someone involved in this work. We will also continue to work with the police, outreach and other organisations striving to make the workplace safer for all concerned.'

SW5

11 Eardley Crescent, Earl's Court, London SW5 9JS

t: 020 7370 0406

f: 020 7244 0037

Office hours: Mon–Fri, 10 am – 5 pm

www.sw5.info

SW5 (formerly Streetwise Youth) is part of the Terrence Higgins Trust. They provide advice, information, help, support and a café primarily to male and transgender sex workers. They take an active interest in all things to do with the sex industry, particularly in London. Their website is invaluable for access to legal information and they regularly post up advice and warnings for all sex workers.

The Poppy Project
2nd Floor, Lincoln House, Kennington Park,
1–3 Brixton Road, London, SW9 6DE
POPPY Project Information Officer – t: 0207 840 7141
f: 0207 840 7139
www.poppy.ik.com
The POPPY Project is a pan-London research and development project working on exiting prostitution and counter trafficking. The POPPY Project also provides accommodation and services to women trafficked into sexual exploitation in the UK..

Base 75
75 Robertson Street, Glasgow G2 8QD
t: 0141 204 3712
f: 0141 221 3498
Office hours: Mon–Fri, 9.30 am – 5 pm
Nightly drop-in: Mon–Fri, 7.30 pm – 11.30pm;
Sun 7.30pm – 10pm
Duty service: Mon–Fri, 2 pm – 5 pm
Medical service: 6 nights per week
Base 75 is the joint health and social care service for prostitutes that operates six nights a week in the red light area of Glasgow.

In Good Company

SCOT-PEP
70 Newhaven Road, Edinburgh EH6 5QG
t: 0131 622 7550
f: 0131 622 7551
voice@scot-pep.org.uk
www.scot-pep.org.uk
SCOT-PEP was set up by and for sex workers and offers non-judgmental advice and support. Our aim is to promote health, dignity and human rights amongst those involved in the sex industry.

Ireland
Women's Health Project
Baggot Street Clinic, 19 Haddington Road, IRL-Dublin 4
t: +353-(0)1 660 21 89
f: +353-(0)1 668 00 50
Office Hours: Wed, 2 pm – 4 pm; Thurs, 8 pm – 10.30 pm
The Women's Health Project is an outreach health service for street workers and brothel workers.

USA
Sex Workers Outreach Project
www.swop-usa.org
A great website with lots of information both in the USA and internationally.

Prostitutes Education Network
www.bayswan.org
A great site for information and links to numerous organi-

Resources

sations, forums and writing by and for sex workers in the USA and internationally.

Sex Workers Project
Urban Justice Center, 666 Broadway, 10th Floor, New York, NY 10012
t: 646 602 5690
f: 212 533 0533
swp@urbanjustice org
www.sexworkersproject.org
In their own words: 'Created in December 2001, the Sex Workers Project is the first program in New York City and in the country to focus on the provision of legal services, legal training, documentation, and policy advocacy for sex workers. Using a harm reduction and human rights model, the SWP protects the rights and safety of sex workers who by choice, circumstance, or coercion remain in the industry.'

Prostitutes of New York (PONY)
PO Box 174, Cooper Station, NYC 10276-0174
t: 212 713 5678
www.bayswan.org/PONY.html
In their own words: 'PONY is a support and advocacy group for all people in the sex industry. We welcome all current or former sex workers, including male, female or TS/TV prostitutes, erotic dancers, nude models, x-rated actors, peep show performers, phone sex workers, S&M/B&D professionals, strippers, madams, and so on. PONY advocates the decriminalisation of prostitution and calls for an end to

illegal police activity – such as street sweeps – in the enforcement of existing laws. PONY provides legal and health referrals to sex workers. Unfortunately, we are unable to provide free legal services. However, our members share information about competent, trustworthy and ethical lawyers who understand the special concerns of sex workers. PONY also encourages members to recommend doctors, therapists and other professionals who provide quality service to sex workers. PONY works to bring all people from different areas of the sex industry together. We encourage all people who sell sex or profit from sex to learn about the diversity of their industry, to promote professional standards within their sector, and to learn more about the history of the world's oldest profession (and its allied industries). PONY encourages you to share your views – and voice your differences – on all issues and topics with other sex workers. PONY (& Friends) is a broader organisation for anyone who supports the rights of sex workers. We welcome the support of johns, feminists and others who care about legal change.'

Canada
Stella
2065 Parthenais Street, Suite 404, Montréal, (Québec) Canada H2K 3T1
t: 1 514 285 1599/1 514 285 8889
f: 1 514 285 2465
stellappp@videotron.ca
www.chezstella.org

Resources

In their own words: 'Founded in 1995 by sex-workers and sympathisers, Stella's goals are: to provide support and information to sex-workers so that they may live in safety and with dignity; to sensitise and educate the public about sex-work and the realities faced by sex workers; to fight discrimination against sex-workers and to promote the decriminalisation of sex work. Stella favours empowerment and solidarity by and amongst sex-workers, since we are committed to the idea that each of us has a place in society, and human rights worth defending. Not only do we run a drop-in centre reserved for sex-workers, but we also produce Bad Tricks and Assaulters Lists included into our monthly Bulletin, a bi-yearly magazine called *ConStellation*, and a growing stock of other useful tools. However, most of our contacts with street-level sex workers, escorts and masseuses and dancers are made through our street work.'

Australia
PROS (Prostitutes Rights Organisation for Sex Workers)
c/o School of Sociology (Att'n: R. Perkins), University of New South Wales, PO Box 1, Kensington 2033, New South Wales
t: 02 6972398

SQWISI,
www.sqwisi.org.au
A great and informative website that was recommended to me by Lyn in Chapter Four. In their own words: 'SQWISI is a community based organisation funded by Queensland

Health, to provide health and information services to the sex industry and the broader community.'

The Magenta Sex Worker Project in Western Australia
www.fpwa-health.org.au/magenta.htm
Magenta provide almost everything from health information and advice to workshops, referrals to government and medical agencies and supplies.

Scarlet Alliance
www.scarletalliance.org.au
In their own words: 'Scarlet Alliance is the Australian Sex Worker Association, the peak body for Sex Worker Organisations/Projects/Groups/Networks representing issues affecting our members and those of Sex Workers at a National Level.'

Sex Workers Outreach Project (SWOP)
69 Abercrombie Street, Chippendale NSW 2008
t: 612 9319 4866
freecall: 1 800 622 902 (Free in NSW)
f: 612 9310 4262
info@swop.org.au
www.swop.org.au
Postal address: PO Box 1354 Strawberry Hills NSW 2012
In their own words: 'SWOP focuses on safety, dignity, diversity and the changing needs of sex industry workers, to foster an environment which enables and affirms individual choices and occupational rights.'

Resources

SWOP in the Northern Territories
t: 89 411 711
www.ntahc.org.au/swop.htm

The South Australian Sex Industry Network
PO Box 7072, Hutt Street, Adelaide SA 5000
t: (08)8334 1666
f: (08) 8363 1046
www.sin.org.au
Office Hours: Tues–Fri, 10 am – 5 pm
Promotes the health, rights and well-being of sex workers. In their own words: 'Our mission is to improve the working lives of sex workers and we are committed to promoting pride and empowerment throughout the sex industry. SIN is funded as a health promotion project that aims to support the current high standards of sexual health among South Australian sex workers. Their services include: Health education and information about safe commercial sex, HIV/AIDS, Hepatitis C, sexual health and other sexually transmitted infections. SIN supplies discounted condoms, lubricant, dams, sponges and gloves to the sex industry through our on site Safe Sex Shop. We also offer free delivery to sex workers and sex industry businesses and Clean Needle Program services. Information, referral, advocacy and support on legal, health, financial and employment issues. As well as producing a magazine and providing training and community education programmes.'

In Good Company

New Zealand
The New Zealand Prostitutes Collective (NZPC)
National Office, PO BOX 11-412, Wellington
t: +64 4382 8791
f: +64 4801 5690
pcdp@globe.co.nz
www.nzpc.org.nz
In their own words: 'The NZPC is an organisation of current and past sex industry workers. They seek an environment that supports the rights of sex industry workers. They advocate at all levels for the rights of sex industry workers. The NZPC lobbies for the repeal of prostitution laws in accordance with the models of decriminalisation. It provides mutual support and information for and by sex workers and educates the public and media about issues affecting sex workers.'

International
Asia Pacific Network of Sex Workers
Concrete House, 57/60 Tiwanon Road, Nonthaburi 11000 Thailand
t: +66 2526 8311
f: +66 2526 3294
http://apnsw.org/apnsw.htm
Working to make sex work safe in Asia and the Pacific.

The International Union Of Sex Workers
PO Box 27465, London SW2 1YA
www.iusw.org

Resources

In their own words, they are demanding and fighting for: 'Decriminalisation of all aspects of sex work involving consenting adults. The right to form and join professional associations or unions. The right to work on the same basis as other independent contractors and employers and to receive the same benefits as other self-employed or contracted workers. No taxation without such rights and representation. Zero tolerance of coercion, violence, sexual abuse, child labour, rape and racism. Legal support for sex workers who want to sue those who exploit their labour. The right to travel across national boundaries and obtain work permits wherever we live. Clean and safe places to work. The right to choose whether to work on our own or co-operatively with other sex workers. The absolute right to say no. Access to training – our jobs require very special skills and professional standards. Access to health clinics where we do not feel stigmatised. Re-training programmes for sex workers who want to leave the industry. An end to social attitudes that stigmatise those who are or have been sex workers.'

The International Sex Worker Foundation for Art, Culture and Education (ISWFACE – pronounced 'ice face')
8801 Cedros Avenue, #7 Panorama City, CA 91402 USA
t: (818) 892 2029 or (818) 892 8109
www.iswface.org
In their own words: 'Our organisation is run by sex workers [current and retired] primarily for sex workers but it is also for *anyone* who wants to learn more about us, including

students, researchers, academics, the media, law enforcement agencies, policy makers and of course, art lovers. An intriguing site with lots of international information.'

Taiwan
Zi Teng
www.ziteng.org.hk
Women's rights, including sex workers in Taiwan. In their own words: 'Zi Teng is a non-governmental organisation formed by people of different working experiences. They are social workers, labour activists, researchers specialising in women studies and church workers etc who care and concern about the interest and basic rights of women. We believe that all women, regardless of their profession, social classes, religion, or races, have the same basic human rights, that they are equal and entitled to fair and equal treatment in the legal and judicial system, that nobody should be oppressed against, that all people should live dignity.'

Drug Addiction
UK
Addaction
67–69 Cowcross Street, London EC1M 6PU
t: 020 7251 5860
www.addaction.org.uk
Addaction is helping individuals and communities to manage the effects of drug and alcohol misuse by providing effective services throughout the UK.

Resources

Lifeline Project Ltd

101–103 Oldham Street, Manchester, Lancashire, M4 1LW

t: 0161 834 7160

www.lifeline.org.uk

A charity fighting and helping many social issues throughout the UK. In their own words: 'Lifeline Project is a non profit making organisation, a registered charity governed by its memorandum and articles of association and a company limited by guarantee. The principal activities of the company are to assist persons and their families and dependents affected by the misuse of drugs and to provide a training and advisory service to persons and organisations who deal with the misuse of drugs and sexually transmitted diseases. Lifeline is a diverse organisation working in a wide range of settings across the breadth of England. We have a significant pool of staff and volunteers who work from our bases in the North West, Yorkshire and the North East. We also work on the streets, in people's homes, in bars and clubs, in prisons and in schools. We work with children and adults, parents and families, people from every ethnic and social background. We work with people who want to stop using drugs and we work with people who want to carry on using drugs. We work with other groups and professionals who want to help drug users; and we work in other areas of the country and other parts of the world to pass on our expertise and experience.'

In Good Company

USA

All the below provide help and advice for the substance addicted:

Safe Harbour Women's Treatment Center
California
t: 949 645 1026/714 323 8294

The Queens Outpatient Substance Abuse
t: 718 849 6300

The Brooklyn Outpatients Substance Abuse
t: 718 383 7200

Australia
The Alcohol & Other Drugs Council
t: Sydney 02 8382 2111 and Melbourne 1800 888 236
Providing help and advice for the substance addicted.

Disabled
UK
The Outsiders Club
t: 020 7354 8291 (please leave a message on the answer phone)
Postal address: The Outsiders, BCM Box Outsiders
London WC1N 3XX (please send a stamped addressed envelope to this address for more information)
Volunteers look after the phone when they can, and always on Thurs 1 – 5 pm.

Resources

Sex and Disability Helpline
Dr Tuppy Owens, BCM Box Lovely, London WC1N 3XX
(please send a stamped addressed envelope with your
enquiry)
t: 0707 499 3527
www.outsiders.org.uk
Mon–Fri, 11am – 7 pm
Outsiders was founded in 1979 by the amazing and vibrant
Dr Tuppy Owens. I have met and worked with her and find
her a total inspiration for all women as well as the disabled
community. In their own words: 'Outsiders is a nationwide,
self-help, community providing regular mailings and
unthreatening events where people meet up and practise
socialising. Members appreciate a club where they are totally
accepted, and some of the most amazing relationships have
been formed. Outsiders is for people who feel isolated
because of social and physical disabilities. The club helps
them gain confidence, make new friends and find partners.
We welcome people of all sexualities, whether they are single, divorced, separated or married, and we discriminate
against no one. Our members appreciate a club where dis-
ability is accepted and people can relax and be themselves.
The first step may be to acknowledge the person's sexuality,
and offer support in asserting their right to a private life, and
seeking love in a society where status normally stems from
good looks and money.'

In Good Company

Domestic Violence
UK
The 24-Hour National Domestic Violence Helpline
PO Box 391, Bristol, BS99 7WS

t: freephone 0808 2000 247

helpline@womensaid.org.uk

This agency will refer to your nearest domestic violence refuge as well as provide support and advice. In their own words: 'Women's Aid Federation of England (Women's Aid) is the national charity working to end domestic violence against women and children. Our mission is to advocate for abused women and children and to ensure their safety by working locally and nationally to: offer support and a place of safety to abused women and children by providing refuges and other services; empower women affected by domestic violence to determine their own lives; recognise and meet the needs of children affected by domestic violence; promote policies and practices to prevent domestic violence; raise awareness of the extent and impact of domestic violence in society. Women's Aid is the national domestic violence charity which co-ordinates and supports an England-wide network of over 300 local projects; providing over 500 refuges, help lines, outreach services and advice centres. Our work is built on almost 30 years of campaigning and developing new responses to domestic violence . . . When all the lines are busy there is a voicemail service that enables callers to leave a message. The voicemail is checked regularly throughout each day and calls are returned as soon as possible.'

Resources

Ireland

Women's Aid

47 Old Cabra Road, IRL-Dublin 7

t: +353-(0)1 868 4721

f: +353-(0)1 868 4722

info@womenaid.ie

Office hours: Mon – Fri, 9 am – 5 pm

Helpline hours: Mon – Sun, 10 AM – 10 pm

Women's Aid offers counselling, streetwork, shelter, workshops, support and information service available to women in abusive relationships.

USA

National Domestic Violence Hotline

t: 1 800 799 SAFE (7233) 1 800 787 3224 (TDD service)

Providing emergency and non-emergency referrals to domestic violence resources in your area (multilingual service available).

Battered Women's Justice Project

t: 1 800 9030111

www.bwjp.org

Providing training, technical assistance and other resources through a partnership of three nationally recognised organisations: Domestic Abuse Intervention Project of Duluth, National Clearinghouse for the Defense of Battered Women and Pennsylvania Coalition Against Domestic Violence.

In Good Company

Catalyst Women's Advocates
t: (530) 895 8476
American Institute on Domestic Violence
2116 Rover Drive, Lake Havasu City, AZ 86403
t: (928) 453 9015
f: (775) 522 9120
info@aidv-usa.com
www.aidv-usa.com
Provides training on domestic violence in the workplace.

Family Violence Prevention Fund
383 Rhode Island Street, Suite 304, San Francisco
CA 94103-5133
 t: 415 252 8900
f: 415 252 8991
fund@fvpf.org
www.fvpf.org
An organisation fighting to end abuse in all situations. In their own words: 'The Family Violence Prevention Fund works to prevent violence within the home, and in the community, to help those whose lives are devastated by violence because everyone has the right to live free of violence. For more than two decades, the Family Violence Prevention Fund (FVPF) has worked to end violence against women and children around the world. Instrumental in developing the landmark Violence Against Women Act passed by Congress in 1994, the FVPF has continued to break new ground by reaching new audiences including men and youth, promoting leadership

Resources

within communities to ensure that violence prevention
efforts become self-sustaining, and transforming the way
health care providers, police, judges, employers and others
address violence.'

Rape Crisis
t: 530 342 7273.

Child Protective Services
t: 1 800 400 0902.

Women's Law Project
125 S. 9th Street, Suite 300, Philadelphia, PA 19107
t: 215 928 9801
f: 215 928 9848
info@womenslawproject.org
The purpose of the Women's Law Project is to provide legal
information, support and assistance to women, men, children and seniors who are victims of domestic violence.
Paralegal interns are available to provide information about
obtaining restraining orders pertaining to domestic violence
and harassment. The interns of the Women's Law Project
work closely with local county and state agencies that are
available to assist the person dealing with domestic violence issues. Interns are available to make referrals to other
private agencies who deal with a wide range of women's
issues.

In Good Company

Australia

Australian Domestic and Family Violence Clearinghouse

University of New South Wales, Sydney, New South Wales 2052

t: 02 9385 2990

f: 02 9385 2993

clearinghouse@unsw.edu.au

www.austdvclearinghouse.unsw.edu.au

A database of domestic violence resources throughout Australia.

New Zealand

Preventing Violence in the Home

195 Khyber Pass Road, PO Box 106 126, Downtown Auckland

Crisisline (24-hour, Auckland only): 09 303 3939

t: 09 303 3938 (for information or resources, call between 9 am and 5 pm, or leave a message and they'll call you)

f: 09 303 0067

enquiries@preventingviolence.org.nz

www.preventingviolence.org.nz

Their mission in their own words: 'To assist people to be safe from domestic violence through 24-hour crisis intervention, education, advocacy, liaison and inter-agency networking. Everyone is entitled to be safe in their homes! Our website can tell you about: Women's experience of domestic violence, and how women can gain safety; men's experience of domestic violence, and what men can do to create non-violent change; preventing violence services available from our agency; training and resources for practitioners to identify when domestic violence is present, and to respond more effectively; training and other links and contacts for information on domestic violence. If you are in danger now, call the Police on III.'

Europe

The Russian Association of Crisis Centres 'Stop Violence'
t: 007 (095) 2509171
rac2women@mtu-net.ru
Campaigning to help women and children suffering from exploitation and abuse.

References

Introduction

1.   Members of the ECP speaking to Rachel Silver in her book *The Girl in Scarlet Heels*, Arrow Books, 1993

2. Guy Palmer, Jane Carr and Peter Kenway, *Monitoring Poverty and Social Exclusion 2004*, Joseph Rowntree Foundation, 2004

3.   www.census.gov/hhes/www/poverty/poverty03/pov03hi.html

4.   ww.abs.gov.au/AUSSTATS/abs%40.nsf/mf/6202.0?Open Document

5.   www.creditaction.org.uk/debtstats.htm

6.   www.abs.gov.au/Ausstats/abs@.nsf/e8ae5488b5988 39cca25682000131612/9ff2997ae0f762d2ca2568a90013934c! OpenDocument

7.   Open Document – Australian Social Trends for the year 2000, www.abs.gov.au/ausstats/abs@.nsf/94713ad445ff142529.

8.   www.creditaction.org.uk

9.   The US Department of Education, www.jbhe.com/vital/ 44_index.html

References

10. http://66.102.9.104/search?q=cache:kJVzsXYw_YcJ: www.ada.org.au/media/documents/News/Submissions/200 3.08.15%2520ADA-Higher%2520Educn%2520submissi on.pdf+Australian+Graduate+debt&hl=en&client=firefox-a (previously 15)

11. American Social Security online, www.ada.org.au/media/ documents/news/submissions/2003.08.15%20ADAHigher% 20Educn%20submission.pdf

12. www.russiansabroad.com/russian_history_157.html

13. 'Domestic Violence's Statistical Factsheet' by Women's Aid Federation of England, Council of Europe, 2002, www.womensaid.org.uk/dv/generaldvfactshindex.htm

14. British Crime Survey, Home Office, July 2002

15. www.womensaid.org.uk/dv/dvfactsh2002.htm

16. www.womensaid.org.uk/dv/

17. The American Institute on Domestic Violence, 2001, www.aidv-usa.com/Statistics.htm

18. Suzanne Snively, Coopers And Lybrand, *The New Zealand Economic Cost of Family Violence*, December 1994

19. www.refuge.org.uk/

20. 'EUROPAP regional reports', www.ex.ac.uk/politics /pol_ data/undergrad/aac/scale.htm

21. ibid

22. The Prostitutes Education Network, www.bayswan.org/ stats.html

23. www.catw-ap.org/facts.htm

24. ibid

25. ibid

In Good Company

Chapter Three: The Reality of Escorting

1. www.mhcs.health.nsw.gov.au/health-public-affairs/mhcs/publications/5500.html
2. www.avert.org
3. www.grindleys.co.uk/jargon_buster.html

Chapter Five: Other Forms of Sex Work

1. www.chatrecruit.com
2. www.telephonesexy.co.uk/unitedstatesusaphoneline services
3. International Watch Foundation, http://www.iwf.org.uk/government/page.101.220.htm
4. www.askmen.com/women/models_250/262_jenna_jameson.html
5. Potterat JJ, Brewer DD, Muth SQ, Rothenberg RB, Woodhouse DE, Muth JB, et al. 'Mortality in a long-term open cohort of prostitute women', *Am J Epidemiol 2004*; 159:778–85, Canadian Medical Association
6. Maggie O'Kane, *Guardian*, Monday 16 September 2002, ww.ixion.demon.co.uk/mediaarchiveseppoct.htm#news10

Chapter Six: The Media and the Law

1. A wonderful female journalist is Zak Jane Keir, who writes for *Desire, Contact UK* and *FRM*
2. The CROSSROADS WOMENS CENTRE, http://ourworld.compuserve.com/homepages/crossroadswomenscentre/ECP/ecphome.htm
3. www.barcouncil.org.uk/document.asp?languageid=1&documentid=2970#ParaLink11

References

4. www.sw5.info/morelaw.htm

5. From a conversation with Niki Adams from the ECP.

6. Cari Mitchell from the ECP, by email

7. www.greenparty.ie/en/in_the–dail/departments/justice_equality_law_reform/16_feb_05_prostitution

8. Timothy J. Gilfoyle, City of Eros: New York City, Prostitution, and the Commercialization of Sex, 790–1920, Norton, 1991; http://college.hmco.com/history/readerscomp/rcah/ html/ah_071700_prostitution.htm

9. www.usdoj.gov/criminal/ceos/prostitution_fedefforts.html

10. http://caselaw.lp.findlaw.com/nycodes/c82/a56.html

11. http://caselaw.lp.findlaw.com/cacodes/pen/261-269.html

12. Catherine Healey, New Zealand Prostitutes Collective, writing in July 2004 for The Summary Response to the government consultation paper on prostitution by the English Collective of Prostitutes

13. www.humantrafficking.org/countries/eap/new_zealand/govt/laws/prostitution_reform03.html

14. www.maxim.org.nz/ri/prbsummary.html

15. ibid

16. www.timbarnett.org.nz/prostitution.htm

17. John Lowman, School of Criminology, Simon Fraser University http://mypage.uniserve.ca/~lowman/ProLaw/prolawcan.htm

18. www.sexwork.com/montreal/law.html

19. www.greenleft.org.au/back/2004/572/572p8b.htm

20. www.wsws.org/articles/2003/jan2003/fran-j30.shtml

Chapter Seven: A Guide for Clients

1. Federal Trade Commission, August 2003 and Celent
Communications via Lafferty Publications,
www.epaynews.com/statistics/fraud.html#34

About the Author

Kay Good founded and runs the escort agency GoodGrrls, for which she won The Erotic Awards Sex Industry Worker of the Year Award 2004. In addition to GoodGrrls, she has managed a dungeon and worked in the areas of domme and sub work, text sex, phone sex, glamour photography and erotic art, and in her teens she briefly worked the hotels of London as a sex worker. She lives in London with her partner and photographic collaborator and a senile cat. In addition to writing and running the escort agency she also photographs, models and builds websites. She is currently working on her next book, which will be a guide to BDSM.